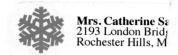

HEALTHFUL
EVOLUTIONS

HEALTHFUL EVOLUTIONS

*Your Guide to
the Prevention and Reversal
of Heart Disease*

DR. MICHAEL DANGOVIAN, DO

OneBreath Publishing

First printing 2017

ISBN: 978-0-9981618-5-3
LCCN: 2016915823

ATTENTION CORPORATIONS, UNIVERSITIES, COLLEGES, AND PROFESSIONAL ORGANIZATIONS: Quantity discounts are available on bulk purchases of this book for educational purposes, gifts, or as premiums for increasing magazine subscriptions or renewals. Special books or book excerpts can also be created to fit specific needs. For information, please contact OneBreath Publishing, 39242 Dequindre Rd., Suite #103, Sterling Heights, MI 48310.

http://www.wellnesstraininginstitute.com

TABLE OF CONTENTS

ACKNOWLEDGMENTS

THIS BOOK IS dedicated to those who know there is a better way. I wrote this book for people who not only crave health and wellness, they desperately want to eliminate the needless suffering from their lives. I have been writing this book in my head for decades. It is no surprise to anyone who has written a book that this is a lengthy process. Not only did it teach me more about health and wellness than I thought I would ever need to know, it taught me a lot about myself. The biggest lesson was that I could not do it without the help of others.

That is why I want to acknowledge a number of people who helped me along the way, beginning with Ellen Daly. Ellen's expertise made it possible to get all those words on the page painlessly. My family was also very important in the creation of this book. I thank my mother and father, Lorraine and Alfred Dangovian, and my children, Marissa and Jake, who provided the inspiration to take on a project like this. They patiently listened to me drone on and on about "The Book," and were required to proofread now and then. I want to thank George Vutetakis who introduced me to Ellen Daley, gave me the name for my SitStandStroll yoga program, and provided me with many of the best meals of my life.

A special thanks goes out to Joan Hill, who would not take no for an answer, and more than anyone made sure that this book became a reality. I first met Joan as a patient and now she is a close personal and family friend. Joan and I spent well over 100 hours, proofreading and editing until it was just right and then some. I would also like to acknowledge Nicole Martin who began as a trusted employee in my wellness institute and is now my business partner. Without Nicole, I am sure I would not have gotten this book over the finish line. And to all of you who I didn't mention, you know who you are, thank you again and again. To be done just plain feels good. I hope you enjoy the read and that it adds something meaningful to your life.

Sincerely,
Dr. Michael Dangovian, DO, FACC

INTRODUCTION

DID YOU KNOW that we have known how to reverse heart disease for over 25 years? Has your doctor or anyone else suggested that it's even possible to reverse heart disease? Perhaps you or someone you love already suffers from heart disease and you are looking for some answers, or you want to stay healthy and do everything possible to prevent this deadly disease. Whatever your motivation for reading this book, I congratulate you on taking this important step on your journey towards claiming responsibility for your health and well-being. Heart disease is a scary thing. It would be so much easier to leave the thinking to the "experts," yet, even with all of their knowledge and modern medicine's major advances, coronary artery disease remains the leading killer of both men and women in the United States. Someone dies every 90 seconds from heart disease! Let's face it—the "experts" have failed us. There is a better way. This book will teach you how to prevent and reverse heart disease.

Healthful Evolutions™ is a simple and powerful program that gives you the tools you need to reverse coronary artery disease by combining the ancient traditions of yoga, the conventional wisdom of medical science, and basic common sense. We will begin by exploring how and why we get heart disease, and then we will learn how to prevent and reverse it in a logical and scientific way. No one should feel left out. Anyone can achieve optimum health and well-being at any stage of life, regardless of their current situation.

Some of my recommendations might surprise you. Be assured that everything is supported by medical and scientific research.

If anyone had told me when I was in medical school that I would one day write a book extolling the benefits of yoga, I would have told them that they were insane. Like most people in those days, I thought of yoga as something exotic and frivolous—good for celebrities like the Beatles, Madonna, or Sting, but not for regular people like me. To even consider that yoga would play a role in reversing a chronic disease process would have been unthinkable. Yet today, not only am I an active proponent of yoga, I consider it essential to living a truly healthy life for the simple reason that no other medical treatment, lifestyle practice, exercise, self-help program, or diet has impacted my life or the lives of my patients more.

As you progress on your journey in Healthful Evolutions you will discover quickly that yoga is not what you think it is. It is so much more than a fitness program. In time, you will come to think of yoga as a new way of being. If you think that sounds far-fetched, you are not alone. I felt exactly the same way when I first started on my own journey more than 30 years ago. I couldn't imagine how twisting my body into crazy positions could save my life, reverse heart disease, or do anything other than aggravate my already aching back. Despite my skepticism, enough scientific evidence was available at the time to convince me to keep an open mind. Ultimately it was my professional and personal experiences that convinced me beyond any doubt that a yoga practice is not only helpful but vital for the healing process to take place.

Unfortunately for many of us, it is only after something goes terribly wrong that we are willing to take a sincere interest in our health. Healthy living takes a set of skills that requires knowledge and practice. Waiting for the problem places us at a disadvantage because it takes time to cultivate the lifestyle skills necessary to heal ourselves.

While it is never too late, clearly now is better than later. Think of this book as a user-friendly manual that gives you the plain and simple truth about how to prevent and reverse heart disease—and so much more. By integrating the basic principles and practices of Healthful Evolutions into your life, you will feel improvement immediately. How can that happen? Because this practice aligns with the natural laws of the universe. It's no mystery why we suffer from our most common problems; our Western lifestyle is the perfect recipe for chronic disease. When you combine the standard American diet, a sedentary lifestyle, lots of stress, long workings hours, and perhaps some smoking and drinking, the natural outcomes are hypertension, obesity, diabetes, and heart disease, as well as many other common chronic diseases. It is the universal laws of nature at work. Just as when we heat water to 212 degrees Fahrenheit, it will boil, so, too, will the body react poorly when we treat it poorly. Once we change the way we live, aligning with the universal laws of nature, our health has to change, and it does so naturally.

The irony is that we are our own worst enemies, because our bodies possess the ability and wisdom to heal themselves. We play the victim, refusing to acknowledge our toxic choices that continuously drain our bodies' resources. When our bodies are continuously engaged in damage control, little energy remains to fuel the healing process. When we take responsibility for our unbalanced lives and choose health, however, our bodies' suppressed healing energies no longer are committed to warding off new problems and finally have a chance to repair the old damage that has accumulated over the years. We improve.

It goes without saying that the more committed you are to Healthful Evolutions, the more dramatic the results will be. Rooted in common sense, these techniques and principles will soon become second nature. You will no longer need to walk on eggshells because you are worried that you are missing something—it's all here, and you will finally be able to live a life of ease, knowing that you are getting well.

It is not so easy to find the answers to health and well-being. When I was 18 years old, I wanted these answers for myself. I asked lots of questions and read what was available to me at the time. All along, I knew something was missing. In college, I went to an internal medicine specialist and asked him what I needed to do to stay healthy. He looked at me like I was crazy and told me to come back when I had a "real problem." When I went to medical school, I thought I would get the answers that I craved, but I was wrong. Now, more than 30 years later, I know the internist was not unwilling to tell me what to do; he simply didn't know because it wasn't part of his training. It wasn't until many years later that I would get the answers to my questions.

My dream, as a physician, is to advance a truly healthy population, as people are living longer than ever before. We already have the technology to make that happen. Just look around any hospital or nursing home. I can't tell you how many patients I have who are living much longer than they ever believed they would. The distressing part is that while they may be happy to be alive, more often than not they are debilitated not from their heart, lungs, or kidneys, but from a failing body structure. They are afflicted with "old age," the classic stooped-over posture that robs them of their vitality and well-being as they progress into their golden years. Healthful Evolutions meets this problem head on, because when we align with the universal laws of nature, our bodies become stronger and lighter. The question is not whether we will live into our 80s and 90s; it's how well we will be living when we are in our 80s, 90s, and beyond. Healing does not occur in a vacuum. Healthful Evolutions addresses all aspects of our health and well-being, including our body structures.

Healthful Evolutions also brings peace of mind. My patients who practice this program are more relaxed and no longer desperate for the newest medical or wellness fad, because not only do they feel better, they *know* they are better. The panic is gone! For the first time they are involved in something that legitimately enhances their lives in a balanced fashion and teaches them how to improve their health and well-being. Finally, they know exactly what to do to give themselves a chance to reduce or eliminate some or all of their medications, reduce hospitalizations, procedures, and surgeries, and feel better than they have in years. And because they are confident that they are doing the right thing, their lives are no longer dominated by fear and anxiety, surrounded by thoughts of their next heart attack.

If that sounds like the way you want to live, then Healthful Evolutions is the program for you. My goal is for you to become your own expert. As you expand your knowledge base and practice these techniques, you will develop a unique and profound awareness and calm. When you hear about the "next big thing," you won't be waylaid by the misinformation we are continuously fed by the medical establishment, media, and even our family and friends.

This book is divided into three parts. Part 1 describes the universal principles upon which all life and this method rests. In Part 2, you will become familiar with the disease process, which will in turn allow you to understand the healing process, so that it is clear to you why you are doing what you are doing. Finally, in Part 3 I present my plan for reversing heart disease, detailing the fundamentals of Healthful Evolutions, as well as SitStandStroll™, my portable yoga practice that you can do during your daily activities, which will propel you on your path to newfound health and well-being.

Healthful Evolutions is not intended to be the last word on how to reverse heart disease; it is a beginning. As you cultivate your skillset and progress on your journey to optimal health and reversal of heart disease, you will encounter unexpected benefits and discover that heart disease is about more than just your heart. Reversing heart disease, or any chronic disease, requires a holistic approach, which by definition involves every aspect of your being. People start the program for one reason, then stay for another. Please be aware that diet and exercise are a huge part of Healthful Evolutions.

Yoga is all encompassing. A healthy diet, exercise, and elimination of toxic behaviors are all considered yoga. The first step in yoga is to cultivate an awareness of ourselves, which means we will be taking a good honest look at how we live our lives on every level. As we become aware of the way we eat, we change the way we eat. As we become aware of how sedentary we are, we exercise more. As we become aware of the sabotaging conversation in our heads, we change the conversation. The list goes on and on. As we cultivate awareness, not only do we see what our options are, we see the wisdom of our options, which gives us the freedom to choose. What you choose is up to you.

Before you begin, write down your goals. It doesn't have to be anything elaborate—just a few of your basic desires. After you are three months into the program, review your list and compare it to what is actually happening in your life. I know you will be pleased.

It's important to note that this book does not endorse any medical changes without the consent of your physician. My hope is that it will inspire you to create a more active partnership with your doctor as you take greater responsibility for your own health.

It's never too late to start. No matter what your current condition or age, you can make a dramatic improvement in your well-being. Welcome to a better life!

Part 1

FOUNDATIONS FOR HEALTH

Chapter 1

Reversing Heart Disease—
and a Whole Lot More

*"We are what we repeatedly do. Excellence then, is not
an act, but a habit."*

—ARISTOTLE

THE KEY TO reversing coronary artery disease is not an expensive
wonder drug, a new procedure, or a risky surgery. It's something
people have been doing for thousands of years: yoga. I have been a
practicing cardiologist since 1991 and led cardiac reversal programs
grounded in yoga for most of my career. I do so because yoga works.
Nothing else—not medicine, surgery, or expensive procedures—has
produced anything close to the benefits I have witnessed in patients
who have integrated yoga into their lives.

The Lifestyle Heart Trial was a groundbreaking study that
definitively proved a yoga-based lifestyle could reverse heart disease.
Conceived by Dr. Dean Ornish—cardiac physician to former
President Bill Clinton and preventative medicine champion—the
study was published in *The Lancet* medical journal in 1990. Prior to
this, virtually no one in the traditional medical community believed
that heart disease, or any other chronic disease, could be reversed.
In *Dr. Dean Ornish's Program for Reversing Heart Disease*, Ornish

describes the path that led to the landmark article that forced the traditional medical establishment to give credence to a nontraditional practice that not only treated, but reversed, a chronic disease.

The Lifestyle Heart Trial had to be very carefully designed because it was undertaken at a time when traditional medicine held a very dim view of yoga, or any other alternative approaches, which tended to be quickly dismissed as quackery. The conventional wisdom at the time was that a chronic disease process might be slowed, but it could never be stopped completely. To believe that a chronic disease process could be reversed, especially with something like yoga, was preposterous. In addition, most doctors had little or no faith in their patients' willingness to sustain the lifestyle changes required by such a program.

"When I first began conducting research in 1977 the idea that coronary heart disease could be reversed was thought to be impossible," writes Ornish. "Equally impossible was the idea that everyday people living in the real world could make and maintain comprehensive changes in diet and lifestyle."

When approaching foundations and government agencies for funding to conduct the study, Ornish was told again and again that his theory was "untestable" because no one would be able to follow the program. He conducted preliminary studies that yielded positive results, but these were quickly attributed to the placebo effect. He met the challenge with The Lifestyle Heart Trial.

For the study, Ornish recruited people already diagnosed with heart disease and divided them into two groups: the usual care group and the yoga group. The usual care group's medical care plan incorporated all of the benefits modern health care could offer at that time: state-of-the-art medications (including statin drugs), dietary modification, education, cardiac rehab, smoking cessation, exercise programs, and so on. The yoga group, on the other hand, was required to eat a nondairy, vegetarian, low-fat, whole-food diet, commit to smoking cessation, exercise, practice yoga, and participate in a cardiac support group on a regular basis. It is important to note that the yoga group did not take any cholesterol-lowering drugs, including statins.

Both groups were required to have a cardiac catheterization or angiogram (a diagnostic test used to measure blockages in the arteries) at the beginning of the study and a second cardiac catheterization one year later. To prevent bias and preserve the integrity of the study, the films from these tests were sent all over the country and interpreted with the aid of a computer model by multiple physicians who had no contact with the patients. The study results showed significant improvement in the disease process one year later in the yoga group and significant worsening of the disease process in the usual care group.

The Lifestyle Heart Trial proved that a yoga-based treatment program, without statins, does indeed reverse heart disease, while the traditional medical model showed continued progression of heart disease despite the addition of cholesterol-lowering medicines. More importantly, not only was there a measured reversal of heart disease in the yoga group, there was a clinical benefit demonstrated by a dramatic reduction of cardiac symptoms. In the usual care group there was a significant worsening of symptoms that accompanied the progression of the subjects' disease.

In addition, Ornish completed a five-year follow-up study where a third cardiac catheterization was performed. The results were consistent with the previous study, with the usual care group showing continued progression of cardiac disease, while the yoga group experienced continued reversal of cardiac disease. What's more, the yoga group had a 50 percent decrease in cardiac events when compared to the usual care group.

You might wonder why you haven't heard more about this landmark research. After all, heart disease afflicts 16.8 million Americans and costs $165 million a year. One would expect that the medical community would have been jumping up and down with glee when Ornish proved that this deadly and costly disease could be reversed. Sadly, this has not been the case. Despite the evidence, the majority of the medical community remains resistant to the concept of reversing heart disease. Some of it might be due to ignorance. Most doctors don't practice yoga or holistic living and tend to treat patients the way they would treat themselves. However, even when doctors are informed, they don't necessarily send patients to this kind of program. The resistance may be financial or stem from fears of medical liability. Some physicians I work with will see me for their own care or refer family, but not patients—a sure sign that they personally recognize the benefits but feel their patients would not be receptive to this unorthodox approach.

Opening My Eyes

I became aware of Ornish's work during my cardiology fellowship training and found it very intriguing. When I was asked to work with a cardiac support group modeled after his program, I was thrilled by the opportunity to observe the effects first hand. Before I knew it, I found myself in a room with about 20 cardiac patients who would dramatically change my approach to medicine forever.

A typical session consisted of one hour of a yoga-based activity such as meditation, stretching, or imagery, one hour of group discussion, and one hour of low-fat, vegan dining. While my original role was as the physician on hand available to answer questions, after the first week, the psychologist who had led the yoga portion bowed out. I assumed the role of leading yoga for the group and we continued to meet weekly for almost three years. In the beginning, I relied on audio recordings, mostly based on imagery and relaxation. In time, I integrated more traditional hatha yoga techniques into the practice.

Perhaps the most important revelation came early on as I discovered the devastating effect heart disease had on these people's lives. I was particularly struck by the way it dominated their thoughts; they acted as if they were living with a ticking time bomb in their chests, not knowing when it would go off but convinced it would. One middle-aged woman complained about the stress of her workplace, as she believed it was the cause of her heart attack and was fearful every time she went to work. Another man refused to go on vacation because he was afraid to get on a plane or be any place where he could not readily access his doctor, even though his heart disease was expertly handled and he was free of symptoms. Many had adopted the role of full-time "vigilantes," on the lookout for any symptom, sensation, or thought that could be related to their hearts. Even the slightest twinge in their chest, neck, or arms could trigger a trip to the emergency room. Articles, books, radio, and television reports on the subject served only to fuel the fire as they were compelled to listen to anything and everything these various media sources had to offer.

As I listened to their stories, I realized how heart disease had decimated their lives and the lives of those around them. Spouses, significant others, and other family members were forced to walk on eggshells to keep from upsetting them. Every activity revolved around their disease process. One person admitted to me privately that sex was not an option due to the fear of causing another event. Some told me that their families had become insensitive and impatient because their doctors had insisted that they were all right and that these concerns were all in their heads. They felt isolated and powerless, and the support group was the first place where they were able to open up about their experiences.

Another unexpected revelation was the disdain the group had for the health care system and their doctors. Almost every participant in the group felt at odds with their personal physician in one way or another, complaining that their doctors did not understand, were not listening, or did not seem to care. Some were embarrassed to admit they called and visited their doctors' offices so frequently that they were not being taken seriously. This made them even more upset, and sometimes hostile. Despite their misgivings, they would not seek the care of other cardiologists, compelled to stay with their current ones because they "knew the case." When my group started complaining about their doctors, it went on and on.

That was when I began to understand what it was like to be a cardiac patient. Many felt betrayed because prior to their diagnosis, they had lived up to their side of the bargain, following all of the rules, eating the right foods, exercising, and adhering to their doctors' instructions. These people were paralyzed, confused, and helpless because, despite all of their efforts, here they were in a cardiac support group trying to make sense of it all.

Remarkably, a dramatic shift began to take place a few weeks into the program, as many of the participants became more positive. They smiled more, looked more relaxed, and complained less. They reported feeling more comfortable at work and travel. For the first time in years they were living without heart disease dominating their thoughts. They were healing, and it wasn't due to a new medication, surgery, or procedure; it was due to a yoga-based therapy. I had never seen anything like this before. People who were previously crippled by their heart disease began to move on with their lives. It was amazing.

Naturally, I wanted a program for my own patients. I set aside late Monday afternoons, and, since November 1995, I have led a two-hour cardiac wellness program that includes one hour of yoga followed by another hour of group support, free of charge. The program has evolved over the years. It was not easy in the beginning, as I naïvely assumed all of my patients would jump at the opportunity to join a class specifically designed to reverse their heart disease. I couldn't have been more wrong. When I started to talk to my patients about the class during office visits, their eyes would glaze over; they would listen politely, and then hope I would never bring it up again. In fact, some chose to go to another heart doctor because they were tired of me trying to convince them to do yoga.

Remember that, in the mid-90s, yoga was just starting to make inroads in the United States. Most people had no idea about or any interest in yoga for their health or anything else. In fact, Ornish was famous mostly because of his low-fat, vegetarian diet, and very few people were aware of the mind-body component of his program. Trying to convince people to do yoga back then was much different than it is today.

In time, many of my patients did come to my program, they stayed, and the outcomes were even better than I had hoped. Before long, there was an average of 20 to 40 participants on any given Monday. I continue to marvel at how well my yoga patients do compared to those who choose not to participate. My yoga patients eat better, stand taller, are stronger, have lower blood pressure and cholesterol levels, are hospitalized less with fewer procedures, take fewer medications, and just plain enjoy life more. The difference is staggering, and I am always thinking of new ways to get more people to attend.

Redefining Yoga: The Creation of SitStandStroll™

I have been leading a cardiac reversal program, in one form or another, for 20 years. This has been, perhaps, one of the greatest privileges of my life. For two hours a week I have been able to share my ideas with hundreds of people over the years. The participants of my yoga group are very appreciative and frequently acknowledge the time I spend with them. I, in turn, acknowledge their support and remind them of the opportunity they have given me to work out my ideas on a weekly basis.

Right from the beginning, people would feel better after attending my Monday program. But feeling good is not enough. The goal is to reverse heart disease. The challenge is helping people understand the practice and, perhaps more importantly, to understand how the practice reverses heart disease. Most of the participants are my patients. Rarely is there anyone in the group that is under 60 years old, and, most weeks, there are only a few who are 90 or older. These are everyday people who just happen to have heart disease and up to that point may have thought that a vegetarian meal was a steak salad.

Most people think of yoga as physical fitness. In the past, an image that might have come to mind was of an emaciated, bearded Indian man contorting himself into a very uncomfortable position. While there is a physical aspect to yoga, in reality, yoga is all encompassing and involves everything that we do. The word yoga means union. When we make the connection between the mind, the body, and the breath, we are practicing yoga.

The practices we traditionally associate with yoga, such as holding certain poses or meditating, are techniques designed to intensify this connection between mind, body, and breath. When this connection becomes our focus, yoga is no longer a fitness regimen. Rather, it is a healing practice. This connection is influenced by literally everything we do.

Healing starts with how we think and act on every level. It is not a once-a-week workout before going to the steakhouse and ordering extra fries. We know that negative thoughts can be harmful to our bodies and our psyches. We know that how we eat, how we exercise, how we relax, and how we feel can impact our physical and mental states. Health depends on everything, and yoga can be applied to everything. That is why when we engage in a meaningful yoga practice we are able to reverse heart disease.

My understanding of yoga has deepened over the years. I have traveled to many workshops and educational programs throughout the country. Each time, I would bring back what I had learned and introduce it in my wellness groups. I would work, week after week, to simplify the practice, breaking it down to its most basic form and language. I learned how to teach yoga without using yoga terminology. The end result is SitStandStroll.

SitStandStroll is a simple and powerful healing practice that anyone can do any time of the day. A truck driver can easily do it while driving across country, as can a grandmother waiting in line at the supermarket. Imagine reversing heart disease while you are sitting at your computer, standing at the bus stop, or walking to the post office. That's why I call it Sit, Stand, Stroll. It will begin to work on the very first day you make it part of your life, and the benefits will continue to accumulate day by day, week by week, and year by year.

We live in a new age of health care. No longer do we merely want to stop the disease process; we want to reverse it. We no longer seek to be disease free; we want to be well. These lofty goals are attainable if you are willing to open up your mind to the reality that it can be done. What is required is that you develop a working model of how our bodies function, learn about your own body's behavior, and then commit to a plan to affect the transformation. I will introduce some of the people with whom I have had the privilege of working and whose lives have changed in unimaginable ways.

You will find many people, including your own doctors, are not aware of the benefits of yoga. That doesn't make what we are talking about untrue, or less valid. As you embark on this journey, have confidence that heart disease is reversible. It has been proven both scientifically as well as in the hearts, minds, and bodies of many patients. Here, you will gain an understanding of the disease process, an understanding of the healing process, and then learn to cultivate these skills to reverse heart disease. Get ready to feel better than you have felt in a very long time.

Chapter 2

A Holistic Approach

"A holistic approach is a recognition of the homogeneity and wholeness of life. Life is not fragmented; it is not divided. It cannot be divided into spiritual and material, individual and collective. We cannot create compartments in life: political, economic, social, environmental. Whatever we do or don't do affects and touches the wholeness, the homogeneity. We are forever organically related to wholeness. We are wholeness, and we move in wholeness."

—VIMALA THAKAR, INDIAN SOCIAL
ACTIVIST AND SPIRITUAL TEACHER

SITSTANDSTROLL IS A holistic approach to health and well-being. The word "holistic" is derived from the Greek *holos*, which means whole. Holos implies the understanding that, as Aristotle said, "The whole is more than the sum of its parts." A holistic healing philosophy, holism, considers all the potential contributing factors to a person's well-being and sees particular ailments within the context of the individual's overall health rather than as isolated events. In other words, everything affects everything. On the surface, holism seems like a very simple concept. However, I became aware of its true meaning by accident.

A Blessing in Disguise

Almost 20 years ago while riding down a steep hill I flipped my mountain bike, landing on my head and seriously injuring my neck and back. Fortunately, I was wearing a helmet; nevertheless, the fall left me in chronic pain, unable to pursue my usual activities such as trail riding, running, in-line skating, and skiing. I couldn't even turn my head to look behind me while driving. A bad back is a bitter pill to swallow 24 hours a day, and I was warned by my physician friends that this would be an issue for the rest of my life.

After my injury, I was unable to do anything strenuous or even low impact, which left very gentle yoga as my only option. Up to that point, I had been doing yoga with my cardiac support group for two or three years on a weekly basis, and while I was always respectful of what could be possible, I had no idea how transformative it could be. When yoga became my primary focus, I began to explore many different styles. It wasn't until many teachers later, when I met Anusara yoga instructor Jamie Allison Turner, however, that everything changed for me. Anusara yoga, a style of yoga developed by John Friend, emphasizes proper body alignment as a major aspect of its practice. Before Jamie, I was always hopeful I would be able to heal my back, but I was not completely sure. I was told more than once, by some very smart people, what had happened to me was unfortunate and I might just have to live with my new condition for the rest of my life. After working with Jamie for just one morning, however, I knew, without a doubt, my back would not only be healed, but it would be better than before. Anusara yoga's emphasis on body alignment gave me a model for healing, and I felt the effects immediately. It just felt right! The clarity of the instruction made it possible for me to heal my back and neck completely. I dedicated myself to the practice by going to workshops all across the United States and working with local yoga instructors. Now I am in the best physical shape of my life and still improving. As it turns out, all of these benefits were accomplished with the same principles Dr. Dean Ornish used to prevent heart disease. Let me explain.

Putting It to Use

As the medical director of cardiac rehabilitation at Beaumont Hospital in Troy, Michigan, I tried to start a cardiac reversal program in addition to my Monday yoga group. My intention was to help participants improve their prognoses by creating a better understanding of their heart disease. What could be better than an opportunity to sit with a board-certified cardiologist and ask him whatever you want to know about your health? If I learned anything from my previous support group, it was that doctors don't listen or spend enough time with their patients.

I was surprised when only a few people attended the first session. I then altered my approach, advertising healthy back and stress reduction programs, which helped to fill the seats. The irony was I taught the same holistic program for back pain and stress reduction that I used to reverse heart disease. I found it puzzling people would choose to attend a healthy back or stress reduction program before a cardiac reversal program, especially when they already had heart disease. The reality is, people devote their time and energy to what's important to them, not necessarily to what's important to their doctor, including this doctor.

We all have different priorities, which focus on our immediate concerns. After a heart attack, the immediate concern is to not have another one. Initially, most patients are extremely motivated and work very hard on "getting it right." However, the trauma of their heart disease soon becomes a distant memory. There might be a family outing, such as a birthday party or a wedding, with limited food options, none of which are heart healthy. At first, when people stray off the path they are very nervous, but then nothing bad happens. Over time they become more relaxed and surmise that they are protected, especially if they are taking their medications faithfully and their cholesterol levels are low. It is even worse for smokers who think they are in control of their addictions. This leads to more indiscretions, and before they know it they are back in the cath lab getting another stent.

My goal for patients is to keep them out of the cath lab forever. When patients resist my offers to have them join in my cardiac wellness program, I appeal to them from the perspective of their overall well-being. I want to know what is important to them. Are they overwhelmed by stress either at home or the workplace? Do they have weight issues? Is their exercise tolerance low? Are they suffering from poor posture? Are they short of breath? Do they have insomnia? Do they have low self-esteem? Do they have back pain? Are they just plain afraid of growing old? Because Healthful Evolutions is a truly holistic healing practice, it addresses all of their concerns, as well as mine. We both get what we want!

Holistic Medicine: What It Is and What It Is Not

Often, people with complex medical problems will walk into my office with bags filled with vitamins and supplements, proclaiming that they are throwing away their prescription drugs once and for all and want to do things "naturally" or "holistically." This is ill-advised and not what holistic healing is all about. Holistic medicine does not distinguish between conventional and nontraditional or alternative therapies; it embraces the best of both worlds.

If you were in a car accident, would you want to rely on some herbs and supplements, or would you seek the aid of the hospital emergency room with all of its resources? There is clearly a time and place for everything. One way to view a holistic philosophy is thinking of it as a blended approach to health care, taking the best from both worlds. Usually, a portion of my patients' treatment plan that you, as the patient, are involved in the healing process, and the holistic practitioner relies on the patient to do his or her part.

I refer to holistic healing as a competitor's sport. It's proactive. It doesn't come in a bottle. You can't buy it online. It's not a procedure, a pill, or a prop. You take part in it. And that's what you are doing right now. You could be watching television, shopping at the mall, or doing any number of things that you like to do. Instead, you are reading this book. You are collecting information that is vital to your well-being. Take credit for this important step.

And, as we enter this new era of health care, with the government and third parties rationing services and dictating the medications doctors can prescribe, there has never been a greater need for us to be our own advocates. No longer can we take the doctor's recommendations at face value. We need to ask questions, investigate independently, and play a larger role in the decision process. The FDA (U.S. Food and Drug Administration) is not always our friend. It is a government agency steeped in politics and red tape, and while its mission may be to protect and serve the public, it often falls short of its intentions. This could be due to conflicts of interest and funding, as well as long-established relationships with many of the pharmaceutical companies, food lobbyists, and government agencies.

A Gallup study showed that "75% of medical costs are due to largely preventable conditions (stress, tobacco use, physical inactivity, and poor food choices)." Our lifestyles are the major cause of our ill health, and this is especially true when it comes to coronary artery disease, which kills more of us than any other disease. If you take the time to understand the cause of the problem, objectively understand your current condition, and then learn and practice a healthy lifestyle, the sky is the limit. You choose your own future. What you do on a day-to-day basis is infinitely more powerful than anything that comes in a bottle. Follow the instructions; feel the difference for yourself.

is rooted in conventional medicine with the intention of cultivating the lifestyle skills that might allow them to discontinue some or all of their medications over time. The benefit is that while they are learning how to live, they remain protected.

Holistic medicine requires a new way of thinking. Conventional medical treatment targets a specific disease process, while the holistic model focuses on creating balance. Thinking of it as a lifestyle is a more accurate description than simply a treatment. We must honestly consider all aspects on how we live. When people ask me what is important, my answer is: everything. That is what a holistic approach is about. The human body actually possesses the ability to heal itself, but it can only do so if one is living a balanced life.

The Laws of Nature

Traditional medicine, with its narrow, fragmented lens, ignores the concept of balance and has little respect for the laws of nature. Just ask the victims of Hurricane Katrina. When you live below the floodplain, sooner or later the levies will break, and they will break again. If we continue to pretend that a fast-food diet is healthy, that we get enough exercise walking up the stairs at work or at home chasing our kids, or that we allocate enough downtime for ourselves in the few days of vacation we take each summer, then we have no right to expect that the levies of health, strength, and vitality will hold.

Medicines and surgery can only do so much. Despite the overwhelming evidence, the traditional approach doesn't fully acknowledge the toll our Western lifestyle has on our health. The Western model assumes medical science will relieve us of our responsibility for our health and provide the solution to our toxic lifestyle so we don't have to change.

When we accept responsibility for our actions it becomes clear that chronic disease is the natural outcome of our toxic lifestyles.

Instead of battling a disease process of our own making, we choose a lifestyle that promotes health. As we align with the laws of nature, we are able to connect to the "ease" necessary to reverse the "dis-ease" process. We surrender to the fact that we are not above the higher principles of the universe.

The traditional medical model is not all bad. If you suffer a traumatic injury in a motor vehicle accident, there is no place you would rather be than in the hospital under the care of specialists. But, when it comes to the prevention and treatment of chronic disease, there is a better way. We need to take ownership for our own health and well-being. The solution might seem awkward at first because it is so different from what we are accustomed to and yet so simple that it seems too good to be true. Believe it or not, in the end, it is just common sense. Live your life one way, you get A; live it another way, you get B. As Aristotle said, "We are what we repeatedly do."

Over the years, I have come to terms with the shortcomings of the traditional medical model. The extraordinary systems of Chinese and Ayurvedic medicine were founded as far back as 5,000 years ago on holistic healing principles. These same ancient principles only recently are being incorporated into the Western medical model, utilizing techniques such as acupuncture, meditation, aroma therapy, and herbal remedies, to name a few. Several major hospital systems have found a place for integrative medical practitioners on their staffs, and many medical schools are making integrative medicine part of their curriculum. Making this paradigm shift in thinking is necessary for true healing to occur.

Choose Your Future

People must take a hands-on approach to their own health and well-being. We have been taught to leave it up to the doctor. No more. The most important thing to understand about a holistic approach is

Healthful Evolutions, when practiced regularly, will make you feel better, often immediately. It cultivates a sense of well-being that is hard to explain but is unmistakable when it happens. In a holistic model, everything about your being is affected because you align with the laws of the universe, and the more you align, the healthier you become. You are the key to your own success.

Take Jessie, for example. Jessie was 55 years old when he suffered a stroke due to a heart rhythm abnormality called atrial fibrillation. He also had coronary artery disease, which required open-heart surgery to bypass several blockages. Following his procedure, I was able to convince Jessie to attend my cardiac wellness program, which he committed to early. Since then, he has continued to practice on a daily basis, working in the more advanced yoga classes, and is living a full and active life. My trouble with Jessie has been convincing him to stay on the few medicines that remain because he feels too good. Now, at 60, he has the vitality of a 25-year-old, and you would never know he had suffered a stroke. Jessie will openly say his stroke was a good thing, because it got him to his current state of health.

If Jessie never had his stroke, he would not have learned how to live. In time, dis-ease would have happened and could have been much worse. Now he is better than ever. As Jessie's case shows, Healthful Evolutions works because it is rooted in education and common sense. It gives you a model for healing in very simple terms, helping you to understand the how and why of what you are doing. You will learn the fundamentals of a holistic lifestyle and how to put them into practice. Holistic healing is a skill and requires practice to reap the benefits. My goal is to make you your own expert so there is no doubt in your mind you are on the right path. You will know it because you will feel better than you have for a long time.

CHAPTER 3

A Healthy Attitude

"Attitude is a little thing that makes a big difference."
—WINSTON CHURCHILL

"Thoughts become things. Choose the good ones."
—MIKE DOOLEY

THE MIND-BODY connection is not a new concept. Experiments in the 1970s and '80s confirmed the connection of the human mind to blood pressure, immunity, and body temperature. Recent advances in neuroscience allow scientists to track alterations of blood flow in the brain with changing moods and various mental states. In his book *The Extraordinary Healing Power of Ordinary Things*, author Larry Dossey describes the discovery of the importance of attitudes, emotions, and beliefs to health as "one of the most significant breakthroughs in twentieth-century medicine." Ironically, this is only a discovery to the narrow, limited viewpoint of Western science. Traditional and indigenous cultures have honored this connection for millennia, but because Western medicine demands a certain kind of proof, it is only in recent decades that mind-body medicine has begun to gain acceptance.

In a holistic healing model, it is clearly understood that our mental and emotional outlooks are important components to our overall health and well-being. As Dossey writes, "Our mental life is not isolated above the clavicles. Each thought and emotion is a message to the rest of the body, mediated by an intricate array of nerve signals, hormones, and various other substances." There is no doubt a healthy attitude is a critical component of the healing process. In fact, it is not just a means to an end, but a part of the end itself. Health is more than a series of lab values—it is a state of mind. Think about this: Can a 55-year-old woman with stage-four ovarian cancer who is expected to live less than six months be truly *healthy*? I would say yes. That doesn't mean you would want to change places with her, but you can appreciate that she could live so fully for those six months that they could be the best six months of her life and the lives of her loved ones.

Being healthy does not imply endless smooth sailing or never having to deal with illness or stress. Rather, it implies that when such difficulties arise, we have the tools to cope with these inevitable issues. The big question is: When you experience such a problem, whether it be health-related or stress-related, where does your mind go? When you encounter a stressful situation, what instinctively comes to mind first? How have you programmed yourself to think? Our mental outlook not only helps determine how we feel, but it also affects our long-term prognosis.

One well-known study looked at the impact of group support on breast cancer patients. The women who participated in a support group were found to have better prognoses than those who did not participate, despite receiving the same medical treatments. There was no exercise involved, just talking. At the time it was a revolutionary concept; now it is a fact that we take for granted.

I have patients who have serious medical issues with very limited prognoses, yet even though they know death might approach at any time, they live each and every day as if it is a party. In contrast, I have many patients who have virtually nothing clinically wrong with them according to the traditional Western medical model yet are miserable and act like they are dying, always worrying about every little ache and pain. Which of these is healthier? Whom would you rather be?

One of my patients, Charlie, has a lot of medical issues, including a severely weakened heart causing him to be chronically short of breath, and end-stage kidney disease requiring him to go to dialysis three times a week. Clearly this is a lot to handle, and most of my patients in similar circumstances would be very depressed. Yet, despite everything, he is one of the happiest people I know and is always telling jokes. No matter what, he never seems to be down.

A healthy attitude is centered on our view of the world and expectations of ourselves and others. In my 20 years as a physician and holistic practitioner, I have witnessed miraculous transformations as people choose health. It happens for so many different reasons. Patients often realize that they are not their diseases; they are actually the same person they were before they became sick. When they stop dwelling on the limitations imposed by their disease and focus their attention on the healing process, everything changes instantaneously. Where there was once despair there is hope. At that exact moment their body chemistry is immediately redefined. Armed with a healthy outlook, they learn to reframe the challenges in a way that creates space for wellness to seep in. In this chapter, I want to share with you some of the key elements I have discovered that can contribute to a healthy attitude, and a healthy body to go with it.

Create Realistic Expectations

A common reason we are unable to follow through on our promises and good intentions is that they are overly ambitious. If you are anything like me, when reading a book like this, you are already planning ahead. You vow never to consume a "bad" piece of food, miss a day of exercise, have a negative thought, etc. In addition, you resolve to give up drinking or smoking forever. And while you are at it, you are going to devote two hours a week to a charitable organization, run three miles a day, and be the best person ever. All commendable intentions, but nearly impossible to achieve.

Unrealistic expectations are a curse that sets us up for failure, which then becomes a source of unhappiness and suffering. Unless we make room for pitfalls, we will always be faced with impossibilities. Not doing so will lead to frustration and can rob you of the opportunity of a lifetime. The goal is great health, not perfection.

The first step in healing is to be kind to yourself. It is never too late to improve your health regardless of your current medical condition. All of us are somewhere in our lives. Many of us believe that it is too late to make any meaningful changes because we are too old, too sick, or it is just too hard. Too often, the conversation in our heads is filled with negative thinking, sapping our energy and enthusiasm. When we buy in to this type of thinking we give up on our dreams. This negative thinking is what creates our attitude. It is as simple as having the glass half full or half empty. We have programmed ourselves to be one way or the other. Once we recognize that it is up to us to choose how we look at the world, then we can follow how we pattern our thoughts.

Eckhart Tolle wrote in his book, *The Power of Now*, "I have no use for the past." These may be the most powerful words ever. Many times we rationalize our negative thoughts as a result of past experiences in our lives. If you are like most people, however, you are listening to the same thoughts over and over again, day after day, week after week, and year after year. This habitual stream of thinking springs up involuntarily, and we accept these thoughts as the truth rather than understanding that they are only thoughts and nothing more. How we view the past is largely up to us, and we have chosen our view, for better or worse. There is also another set of unrealistic expectations worth addressing. If your expectation is that you will never die, this will be a problem. On the surface, it may sound ridiculous for anyone to expect to live forever, but I can assure you most of my patients have not made room in their minds for the fact that they will die. Many people feel they are indestructible, no matter how old they are or how unhealthy the lifestyles they lead. So, when they develop conditions like hypertension, coronary artery disease, diabetes, or cancer, their expectation is that anything and everything should be easily fixed with a procedure or a pill. They are often outraged there is not a simple medical cure at hand. Healthful Evolutions addresses these issues by cultivating perspective. Many spiritual traditions have practices that ask practitioners to visualize their own death. This might sound silly, but Western society has shielded us from this natural process for years. In the not-so-distant past, people would routinely die at home, and the wake was held with the deceased laid out on the dining room table. In this age of modern medicine, because few die at home, we have become disconnected from the process of death. When we have elderly or extremely ill family members in the hospital, much needless suffering results from futile treatments and tests because neither the family nor the patient can come to terms with the grave prognosis that is presented to them. For most, no matter how sick they are, they view it as giving up on life, failing, or being a quitter. The tragedy is how much quality time is wasted due to fear of death and the unknown—time that could be spent with one's loved ones, in a peaceful and dignified setting. Most people are either afraid or don't want to make that decision for another family member, but I believe it is often because they haven't come to terms with the reality of death for themselves.

I frequently ask patients if they are worried about dying. The question will catch them off guard, and most times they will tell me that they are. My response is, "Don't worry, you will! And now that we've established that fact, let's go about the task of living." This is a very important teaching and a crucial element in Healthful Evolutions. Before we can live, we need to understand that we must die.

One of my favorite inspirational stories is about a man with metastatic pancreatic cancer who, when given the grim prognosis, decided that instead of subjecting himself to the usual surgeries and chemotherapy, he would quit his job and sail around the world. He outlived his prognosis by 200 percent and had the time of his life. On his deathbed, he confided it was worth it to have finally lived. No chemo, no treatment, just doing what he loved. He needed to be told he was going to die before he decided to live.

Our goal is to live the best life possible for as long as possible. Let's have fun and know that today is going to be the best day ever, every day. And, while we are at it, we are going to reverse our heart disease and other chronic medical conditions. That is our short-term and long-term goal. We are not going to let unrealistic expectations like immortality or never suffering an illness get in the way of what we truly desire, and we are not going to let negative thinking get in the way either.

Whether you want to improve your posture, lose weight, reverse your heart disease, or reduce or eliminate your dependency on some or all of your medications, Healthful Evolutions can help get you there. All of these things can happen, over time. Keep in mind what your current state of health is before you decide you have succeeded or failed. What if success is simply feeling good and being happy? Would you settle for that? And what if feeling good and being happy kept you motivated and committed to a healthy lifestyle, but it took four or five years to attain the seemingly unattainable? So much is possible when you feel good.

There will be bumps in the road, and you may deviate from the program in one way or another. The reason for this is simply that you are a human being. We are imperfect and sometimes inconsistent. My hope is you will leave a lot of room for compassion—particularly for yourself—as you embark on this incredible journey. Your goal for yourself, through the steps in this book, is to reverse heart disease. My goal for you is to live your best life possible. You can do this!

You are going to feel better than you have in years, perhaps as far back as your childhood. As you cultivate these lifestyle skills, you will understand this more than you know.

When you deviate from the program, it doesn't mean you have failed. It just means that you made a different choice. The correct choice is still available—you just need to choose it the next time. At first, it will be easy. I call this the honeymoon period. You feel good immediately, and you can't imagine that you would ever go back to your old habits. But then, because you feel good, you skip a day or two, perhaps make poor dietary choices because you are on vacation or visiting with friends and family, and you really don't feel too bad because of all the work you have already done. A few more days, weeks, or months later, you're back to your old ways completely.

The beauty of Healthful Evolutions is that, even though you strayed, when you return to the program's principles, it will feel better than ever because of the time and effort you have already put in. I'm not recommending you stray, but I am encouraging you to leave room for your humanness to surface every once in a while and not beat yourself up because of it. Just recognize it and return to the program. Make a better choice today. Be good to yourself.

Those who stay on the program for any extended period of time discover quickly that the benefits are cumulative. Each day is better than the one before, and over time you will experience things you never thought possible. That is why, even though you have set a goal, it is also important to open your mind to unexpected possibilities beyond your goal. What if you found out what you thought you wanted wasn't really what you wanted at all? Our health goals might start out with the relief of immediate problems or more cosmetic concerns about how we look. But ask yourself again: What is it that you really, truly want in your life? This may be different from what you think you want right now. There's no need to worry; you do not have to have all of the answers right now. Simply allow the question to remain open, even as you set and achieve your short-term goals. Ask yourself what it would take to make each and every day magical.

Good Intentions Are Not Enough

I would really like to tell you all you need to do is buy this book, read it once, and everything will automatically occur without any further effort. I probably could sell a lot of books if that were true. What is clear, however, is there are no miracle cures or drugs that can take care of all of our woes, especially regarding how to live a healthful life. In order to succeed, we need more than good intentions. I can't tell you how many patients I have who understand exactly what they need to do but somehow feel that, because they understand, they don't need to actually do any of it. I know this sounds illogical, but it is all too common, even among very smart and successful people.

I have been confused for years by the fact that so many of my patients who are successful and accomplished in so many aspects of their lives are unable or unwilling to make simple common-sense lifestyle choices for the sake of their own health. How do we explain the CEO of a multimillion-dollar company who manages international mergers and corporate high finance impeccably yet has allowed his own body to become extremely overweight, causing hypertension, heart disease, and diabetes? How can someone so smart and successful fail to connect the dots between his lifestyle choices and the looming prospect of being placed on dialysis because his kidneys are failing? How could he really believe that changing to diet pop instead of regular pop will be enough to correct his problem? If he ran his company the way he takes care of his body, he would be bankrupt by now.

It is my belief that we all have issues like this—areas in which we know better but seem irrationally unable to act on what we know. Some are more visible than others, such as obesity, while others are hidden, such as financial incompetence or private addictions. We need to have compassion for each individual, but we also need to have compassion for ourselves. We need to recognize that it is within our power to change for the better.

We need to commit if we are to reap the benefits of SitStandStroll. Many of us promise to change our ways and improve our health. Unfortunately, while all of us possess the ability to succeed, adopting a healthful lifestyle takes more than just good intentions. It takes a real dedication to the process, and the truth is that most fail. It's the same way with just about everything else in life. We don't plan to become sick; it's something that seems unexpected but actually, inevitably, occurs over time. Either we don't know or don't believe we are placing ourselves at risk.

We do the same thing with our finances. We don't plan to fail but get into debt anyway. We assume we are not going to make the same mistakes everyone else has. When we are young and making a good living we want to be comfortable. Intellectually, we know we have to save for our retirement, and we intend to do so in time, but the future comes faster than we think. The few who really succeed are those who have an effective plan in place early on, commit to the process, and follow through with action. No matter how smart we are, we do not instantly become financially independent just because we know we need to save our money, and we do not become healthy just because we know we need to eat well and exercise. We actually have to eat well and exercise. We hold the keys to our future.

The hard truth is that everything changes. We are either getting better, or we are getting worse. We can know everything there is to know and still suffer from preventable, lifestyle-induced diseases. We may have very sincerely intended to do the right thing, but we never did and now feel it is too late to get that pristine result we idealized in the past. We rationalize: If we can never achieve that ideal, why do it at all? Some will add that, in fact, they like their lives exactly as they are and stubbornly refuse to compromise their unhealthy ways. The problem is they have a chronic progressive disease, which means their condition will worsen. A middle-aged well-controlled diabetic who is just on oral medications often takes comfort that he is only on pills and not "on the needle" yet, and he behaves as if he is not truly diabetic. The sad truth is, if he does not make any significant changes, he may very well progress to needing insulin at some point and, worse than that, suffer from any of the multiple issues that go along with diabetes, such as kidney failure requiring dialysis, blindness, erectile dysfunction, neuropathy, heart attacks, strokes, and amputations. Unfortunately, it's hard to help people understand how truly miserable their lives can become until they have "a real problem." The sad truth is the condition could have been reversed, and a pristine opportunity has slipped by.

Make Informed, Conscious Choices

Remember, yoga is really about making good choices over and over again. Decisions about lifestyle take place on many different levels. Perhaps the decision on how deep you want to delve into your own being needs to be made first. You can change superficial things, and these will make a difference, but with a limited scope. More meaningful changes will lead to bigger results. Some will feel victimized by the bad choices they made in the past, as if God or the universe has it in for them. The reality is, it's not personal. However, I do believe there is a code of justice in the universe. It's very simple. Our choices have consequences. When we make a decision, we make it for better or worse. Some choices we make have positive consequences, and others have negative consequences. As we become more aware, we understand what is helpful and what is not. If we decide to smoke, for example, we know the consequences of that choice. As adults we have the right to make that choice, but we can also choose not to smoke. If we choose to do so knowing it is a health hazard, that doesn't make us a bad person, but we will reap the consequences.

In Western culture, we tend to want to impose our preferred lifestyle on the universe and expect the universe to comply. We think we deserve to do whatever we want to do, within certain agreed-upon moral limits. But the universe doesn't really work that way. Eastern cultures call this the law of karma. In Western society, we call it getting what you deserve. In Western religious traditions, there tends to be a connotation of guilt and punishment, often associated with a judgmental deity. In the Eastern traditions, karma is simply seen as a natural consequence of choices and actions, a cycle of cause and effect that is woven into the fabric of the universe. Either way, your choices have consequences. Choose wisely and you will live well.

When it comes to health, it is important to respect the law of cause and effect and take responsibility for your own choices. We are not cursed simply because we can no longer eat a hamburger and fries three times a week and remain healthy. The negative consequences are actually quite natural and to be expected. Instead, let us feel blessed that we now know the difference and celebrate all of the healthy foods that are available to us. We have the choice to be happy.

Remember, physicians are not all-powerful deities, nor are they your parents. Physicians can help to make rules for you, but it is not their responsibility to check on you every day and punish you if you don't comply. Physicians are merely consultants whom you pay for their opinions. It is up to you to accept or reject any of the recommendations they make. Many of my patients ask me: What choice do I have? The reality is, my patients hold the power, and the choice is and always has been theirs to make. I can't make anybody do anything they don't want to do. As I get older, I am becoming more comfortable in accepting that concept.

Disease is not a punishment. It is the logical outcome of the way we choose to live our lives. It's time to grow up and take ownership of our actions. There is so much talk about the obesity epidemic in America, as if it were a mysterious disease for which no one could figure out a cause. Is there any real mystery as to how this has happened? I don't think so. We continue to have these deep philosophical discussions as to why it is so pervasive. Perhaps we should look at the obvious and simply conclude we are consuming too much bad food and not exercising enough. Instinctively, we know this to be true. The obesity rate in the United States is one of the highest in the world: a massive 33 percent and rising. Two-thirds of people in the United States are either overweight or obese. A 2009 Gallup poll of 400,000 Americans found only 27 percent got the recommended 30 minutes of exercise five days a week. We are not victims when we create our own conditions. No surprise, no judgment; that's just the way it is. And there are no shortcuts. Your behavior directly impacts your health and well-being. It's not personal; it's just the way it is.

If we don't know any better, we really can't be held accountable, but once we know what is happening then it is a completely different story. While I am asking you to take responsibility for your choices, I don't mean to blame or judge you for where you are now. A lot of it is not your fault. We have all been misled by a society that cares little for "inner work." Our culture is shortsighted and panders to our desire for pleasure and comfort. Our culture is also heavily influenced by big business, and there is a lot of misinformation designed to convince you that many unhealthy foods and habits are truly healthy.

Don't spend too much time ruminating over your past mistakes, as it will only make you miserable. It doesn't mean you shouldn't examine the past, but be careful not to live in it. Consider that what happened was exactly what you needed to get you here today, and it is all about to change for the better.

Be Patient

It is ironic that when we are sick we call ourselves "patients," yet patience is a virtue that few of us seem to possess. As a doctor, I find it frustrating how many people give up when they have barely started simply because they expect miraculous results too soon. With chronic conditions like heart disease, it takes us decades to feel the effects. How much time are you willing to invest for a lifetime of health after spending so many years becoming ill? Healing is a process, and a lifelong process at that. As you integrate the practices of SitStandStroll into your lifestyle, they will become part of your being. Remember, we are not just seeking change; we are seeking transformation. We are going for the gold ring! With practice, this process will become second nature to you. This means you will start to do it instinctively, without thinking, and when you are not doing it, you will feel as if something's wrong, which you will sense quickly and be able to correct naturally.

This brings us back to the matter of expectations. The Buddha told us expectations create suffering. Let's remind ourselves everything changes and, in this case, many of the positive changes that will occur for you will be unexpected. Imagine being Christopher Columbus sailing across the Atlantic for the first time when he left on his journey looking to land in India. He had no idea when he was going to land, and what he found was certainly not what he expected, but it was nevertheless extraordinary. Imagine if he had given up after a few days at sea, frustrated because he wasn't getting anywhere fast enough, and turned around. Have patience, and not only will you get the results you want, you may get results you couldn't possibly imagine.

Have Fun and Be Kind to Yourself

Again, it is important to have fun with this. That is one of the most important choices you can make as you embark on your journey to health. Most of us wouldn't immediately connect health matters with fun, but there is good reason to make the connection. Beginning this program may be the first proactive thing you have done for yourself in years. Don't you deserve to reward yourself while improving your health and well-being? While the importance, magnitude, and gravity of the reasons you have for pursuing this program may be at the forefront of your thinking, it's the fun that will keep you going. What if your job was your absolute favorite pastime? You would have a lot more motivation to go to work. Shouldn't it be this way with our health?

I remember when I first began on my own path and started learning yoga. Often I would struggle and strain to learn a new concept or pose, thinking the faster and harder I worked, the quicker the results would come. Ironically, this caused my body to stiffen due to my overzealousness and slowed my progress significantly. In fact, I had a tendency to over-think everything. It was only when I finally relaxed and began to enjoy the practice that my mind, body, and heart opened up, I started to have fun, and then the instructions began to make sense. The less I struggled with the instruction, the easier it was to execute the command. So when you find yourself straining and struggling (and you surely will at some point on the path), surrender to the fact that this is a process, it takes time, and reaffirm you are doing it in the spirit of exploration, discovery, and fun.

Again, above all else, be kind and loving towards yourself on your mission. Try not to get down on or belittle yourself should you not immediately see the results you want. By maintaining a positive attitude, you will keep your practice light and free by directing your love and kindness inward. What I often notice is how much latitude we grant our children's missteps and how little room for error we grant ourselves. If we make a mistake, we think about it over and over again, but if our child or grandchild has an issue, we become very compassionate and display a tremendous amount of understanding. Invoke the image of yourself about to learn what you have wanted to know for your entire life; you have all of the time in the world to do it. And having fun in the process is the key to success.

Many of my teachers have told me the most important yoga pose is to smile. Try to smile a lot. Embrace that attitude now as you embark on this journey, as it is the foundation for your health. Yee-hah!

PART 2

UNDERSTANDING DISEASE, UNDERSTANDING HEALING

CHAPTER 4

What Is Health?

"Health is a state of complete harmony of the body, mind, and spirit."

—B.K.S. IYENGAR

IN 1946, THE World Health Organization took the bold step of offering a broad definition of health, describing it as "a state of complete physical, mental, and social well-being and not merely the absence of disease or infirmity." It surprises people when they hear this for the first time because most believe that in order to be healthy, you have to be free of disease. The reality is everyone will have to deal with health issues sooner or later. Being healthy does not mean being free from all illness, but it can imply you are free of dis-ease.

If I run a small business, or even a large company, and I am making a great profit, is my company healthy? One might think so, but then a problem arises. If my company is healthy, it will be able to withstand whatever issue comes along, and while I might not be as profitable for the short term, my company will recover and be stronger in the long term. If my company is unhealthy, it will collapse at the first sign of trouble. Even the largest and most profitable companies in the world face obstacles.

Now, take the example of a 55-year-old man who has exercised his whole life. He has run several marathons over the years, eaten what he believes to be a balanced diet, doesn't smoke, and has had a few glasses of red wine with dinner each week. All of a sudden he developed cancer of the tongue. After careful consideration, he went for surgery to remove a small part of his tongue, followed by short courses of chemotherapy and radiation. He returned to my office and complained he doesn't feel up to snuff only eight weeks post-procedure. Mind you, he had just played a round of golf a few days prior to his appointment with me. He confided that his biggest issue was concern that his current diet was going to lead to coronary artery disease because eggs, milk, and meat went down the easiest after his surgery. I asked him if every one of his health care providers had told him that he was doing tremendously well. He responded that they all had, in fact, told him his recovery has been nothing short of remarkable. So I asked him what it was that he expected. He merely said he expected to be better, faster. I reminded him it had only been eight weeks and reassured him that we would work out his diet over time.

I then changed the discussion, asking him to look for the hidden blessing in all of what had happened. I explained that all of these years he had been "in training" for just such an instance. Since he had already developed excellent lifestyle skills, he was able to integrate this tragedy into his life with ease and grace. Remember, he had just finished 18 holes of golf a few days earlier. Clearly my statement caught him by surprise.

Dis-ease, as I will discuss in the next chapter, literally means you are out of ease, or out of balance. Often an illness or injury causes this lack of balance, but this does not have to be the case. In fact, by coming to terms with an illness or injury on a profound level, you live a life of balance and ease. While you are not free of the illness, I would argue that you are healthy. You have integrated the illness into your being in such a way that you found the hidden blessing inside a dark experience in your life. Health is about having a stable foundation so when you do encounter challenges in your life, you can integrate them into your being and remain balanced and at ease.

An integrated, whole, healthy person lives life to the fullest no matter what the situation. More than anything, that is what I want for every person who comes to me, whether they are reading this book, sitting down in my office, or attending one of my workshops. In order to achieve this, I want you to accept what is happening and what you know right now. You need to stop seeking the "miracle shortcut" to all of your problems. This doesn't mean you stop your quest to improve your condition, but it does mean you should stop worrying so much about what you might be missing. Continue in the spirit of exploration. Imagine if you could pursue your own health and well-being with the same curiosity, innocence, and zest for life that a child brings to his first nature walk.

Life is a beautiful thing. It is a gift we have been given to use in any way we desire. By altering our perceptions, we change our reality. It doesn't necessarily mean we are free from coronary artery disease, hypertension, arthritis, or any other illness. It means how we handle these illnesses and what we do with our lives is totally up to us. How do we change our reality? Energy!

Energy and the Breath

It is a scientific fact that everything in the universe is made up of energy. That's the whole point of Albert Einstein's famous equation, E=MC2, which explains how mass and energy can be changed into each other. You may find it a little hard to get your head around that concept, however. When you look at the world around you—the solid ground under your feet, the trees swaying in the breeze, the car driving by, the apartment building towering above you—it may be difficult to see all these solid objects as being made of energy. But they are.

So let's approach it a different way. Can you accept that everything in the universe is made up of atoms? Atoms are the basic building blocks in nature. The composition of an atom is familiar to most of us, and it is common knowledge that everything in the universe is composed of atoms. The floor, the ceiling, our flesh, and the air are all composed of atoms. An atom has a nucleus made up of protons and neutrons with electrons orbiting around it, the same way the planets in our solar system orbit around the sun. Realize that the planets never stop orbiting the sun, and if they did the results would be catastrophic. So if everything is made up of atoms, and these atoms have orbiting electrons moving around the nucleus at all times, that means there is perpetual movement in literally everything in the universe, including the chair you are sitting on right now.

This concept of perpetual movement is easier to appreciate when considering things like water, air, plants, or animals, but what about the floor beneath your feet, the stones in your driveway, or the fence surrounding your backyard? Those are made up of atoms, too. Are they moving? You bet they are. Even though you can't see it or feel it, it's important to understand that the movement is there. This imperceptible movement is commonly called "vibrational energy," and it is something you can learn to tune in to. Everything has its own vibrational frequency. Light vibrates at a very high frequency, while a rock vibrates at a very low frequency. As living beings age, they begin to vibrate at a lower frequency. No two things in nature have the same vibrational energy.

So what does that mean for you, your body, your health, and your heart? It means that if there is energy and movement in everything, there is energy and movement in all of the cells and structures in your body, too. You can learn how to understand and, more importantly, how to experience this energy flow in your body and then allow it to work for you.

Energy Flows in the Body

Another way to think about vibrational energy is as a rhythm. Rhythms are very important to our health. There are healthy rhythms and unhealthy rhythms in our body. When we are in a healthy rhythm we feel good. An example of this is your heartbeat. Place your hand on your chest and you will feel its powerful, reassuring rhythm. But if you've ever had a heart attack, or even experienced palpitations, you will know just how bad it feels when that rhythm is interrupted. Rhythms in the body are simply energy flowing in a specific way. There are many different rhythms, or energy flows, in the body. Feel how your breath moves in and out of your body. This is an energy flow. There are other energy flows you may be less aware of: the flow of blood through your arteries and veins; your gastrointestinal tract; your nervous system; your musculoskeletal system; your skin. One of the most overlooked energy flows is the stream of thoughts as they flow in and out of your mind. If we can agree there are a multitude of energy flows in our bodies and minds, it stands to reason the flows can be either beneficial or harmful to our health.

Think of an energy flow in nature: a river that flows from a high mountain spring down to the ocean below. When that river is flowing smoothly, the water stays fresh, travelers can use it to move by boat from one place to another, trade can flourish, and the surrounding land can be irrigated by tributaries to the river, supporting vibrant farming communities and industries. Fish can migrate to their breeding grounds, and birds and animals that prey on those fish can find food, enabling them in turn to feed their young. The cycles of nature and culture can continue, nourished by the river's flow. If that flow becomes sluggish, however, if water levels fall due to drought, the river becomes stagnant, the crops die, the fish cannot migrate, and the health of the ecosystem is compromised. On the other hand, if the flow becomes overpowering, swelled by floods, it can also have catastrophic consequences for the land, the fish, birds and other animals, and the communities that depend on the river.

The same principle applies to the energy flows in your body. An obvious example is the gastrointestinal tract. When you eat something, the food goes in one end and comes out the other. How you feel during the process depends on the flow of energy in your gut. If there is a healthy flow, then you will feel energized by the food. You will feel light, and the food will pass through your body providing nourishment and vitality without any discomfort. If your gut is having a bad day, however, you might get abdominal cramping or nausea, you might vomit, have diarrhea, constipation, and many other unpleasant symptoms. If this is a chronic problem you might develop gastritis, an ulcer, a blockage, infections, or even certain types of cancer. What affects the flow of energy in your gastrointestinal tract? Everything. What you eat, what you do or don't do, what you think, and many more factors. Let me explain.

There are many, many parts of our lifestyle that affect our energy flows. I like to divide these into draining (toxic) and energizing (nontoxic) behaviors. Eating unhealthy food, a draining behavior, will make you feel bad. If you eat healthy food, you will feel energized. If you eat too much or too little food, you will feel poorly. If you don't exercise or are very sedentary, you will feel bad. If you are active, you will feel good. If you are too active, you won't feel well. If you are stressed and constantly thinking negative thoughts, you will feel bad. If you change your attitude and replace the negative thoughts with positive thoughts, you will feel better. In the end, it's all a matter of simple cause and effect.

I am sure you have observed this in the people around you. You are standing in line at coffee shop and the person in front of you, who is obviously overweight and unhealthy, orders a grande mocha with whipped cream. Automatically, the thought runs through your mind, "No wonder he is in such bad shape…" Your coworker who constantly complains about everything calls in sick yet again, and you can't help but feel that there is a connection between her endless negativity and griping and her poor health. An elderly relative is diagnosed with lung cancer, and immediately you recall his endless chain-smoking on the front porch after dinner each night. We have an instinctive sense of the difference between healthy, energizing behaviors, and toxic, draining ones. After all, most of it is just common sense. Unfortunately, however, it is much easier to perceive the direct and obvious connections between cause and effect when you are looking at other people than it is when you are looking at yourself.

My point at this moment is not to tell you what is good or not good for you to eat, do, or think. That is something you will learn to discern for yourself as you cultivate greater awareness and engagement with your own body. First, you need to understand that the disease process is due to a disruption of a healthy energy flow. In medicine we refer to this as dysfunctional. Dysfunctional rhythms lead to disease.

Once you are able to consciously connect with the energy currents within yourself, you can harmonize that inner energy and learn how to work with it. This is a skill that must be learned, just as a child who is learning to play a musical instrument for the first time must begin by learning scales—practicing slowly at first, and then faster. At first the youngster complains about how boring it is to endlessly practice, but once these scales are mastered, the new skills bring about a newfound freedom and the capacity to play.

As you learn to recognize and experience the different energy flows within your body, you will also discover an even deeper flow. You will find that within us there is a force, if you will, that is continuously pulsing through our bodies, a current of energy that essentially propels us through the day. That flow of energy is the true you—your essence. Some people call it the life-force, the elan vital. The wisdom traditions of the East call it Qi (pronounced chee), prana, or kundalini. When this force, or energy, is diverted, like the river getting trapped in a stagnant eddy, it results in imbalance and dis-ease. When it is allowed to pulsate unimpeded, we are blessed with optimal health and well-being.

Understanding Health

This chapter began with a question: What is health? The answer may have been very different than you imagined. As you begin to play with the process, you will come to realize how experiencing energy as it flows in our bodies and in nature will bring you to a deeper understanding of what health is. When these energy flows align with the universal laws of nature, we are liberated and begin to feel a sense of wholeness. The underlying unease that keeps us always looking for that something else that was missing will fade. You will develop a deep ease of being, which is the ultimate antidote to the dis-ease that plagues so many of us. Once again, you may still fall ill at times, or have to contend with the injuries and physical challenges that are an inevitable part of an engaged human life. However, when the energy flows in your body are working in harmony with the laws of nature and you encounter these obstacles, the healing process will be able to work naturally, and you will be able to integrate these inevitable life experiences into your being. Your health—your wholeness—gives you the energy to heal.

Although you may not be aware of it, our bodies have the ability to heal themselves. The novelist and painter Henry Miller understood this when he wrote, "Our own physical body possesses a wisdom which we who inhabit the body lack. We give it orders which make no sense." The healing process, therefore, could be seen as a practice of learning how to inhabit our bodies more wisely, with greater awareness, so that the choices we make—the orders we give to our bodies about what to eat, when to sleep, when to move—begin to make sense. Consider that each and every cell in our body possesses its own complement of DNA, and therefore each cell has the ability to act on its own. If we can, through awareness and conscious engagement, remove the obstacles to our natural healing energy and respect the inherent wisdom from within, we will find that doing the "right" thing becomes easier and easier. It begins to feel natural and it should—being healthy is what our bodies instinctively strive for.

Healthful Evolutions has been designed to help us experience the true nature of our existence so we can create a strong foundation and strike the balance with nature that we crave. It turns out the only way to counter disease is with ease. Through this practice, you will cultivate a deep connection with your inner healing energy, which is required to achieve a state of ease.

CHAPTER 5

What Is Disease?

"Sickness is the vengeance of nature for the violation of her laws."

—CHARLES SIMMONS

THE WORD DISEASE comes from the Middle English disese, which is derived from the Anglo-French desaise. Its two syllables are dis-, meaning bad, and ease. So disease does not really mean unhealthy; it means out of ease, or out of balance. Expanding on the theme we explored in the previous chapter, it implies that the energy flows of our body are out of balance. When we develop a chronic disease process such as hypertension, coronary artery disease, or diabetes, it is the result of a long-standing imbalance within our own bodies and between us and our environment. Ultimately, what we are trying to do is restore a state of ease with energy-balancing practices so that the body's energies flow in a healthy way, in alignment with the universal laws of nature.

My goal as a physician is to help people develop a deep understanding of their current condition so that preexisting chronic diseases, such as heart disease or diabetes, or structural problems, such as degenerative disc disease, become less of a mystery. This insight is crucial to the process of allowing patients to become effective partners in healing and disease prevention. The words "healing" and "disease prevention" take on a whole new meaning, because it becomes crystal clear to the patient what is beneficial and what is deleterious to their health and well-being.

If you truly understand the principles of disease, you can then act as an expert on your own behalf. I am not saying you don't need the expert help of those who have gone through decades of medical study, training, and hands-on experience in health care but that you can come to your doctors knowing your own body and understand the underlying principles of your condition.

As I have explained, there is an inner healing energy within each and every one of us. When I tell people this, often the response is, "Well, if that's true, then let's see it. Bring it on! I want to be healed." But that is easier said than done. Why doesn't healing just happen on its own? What is that healing energy doing? Come out, come out, wherever you are! The fact is that your body is working overtime dealing with the toxicity that has accumulated in it over the years. This toxicity creates an imbalance, which leads to chronic disease and the lack of vitality that so many of us feel.

How do we become toxic? The toxicities occur on many different levels. First, we are surrounded by environmental pollutants in the air, water, and land. Then, there are chemical exposures in the environment and our food. There are toxins that we ingest into our own bodies because of poor food choices, subjecting our digestive systems to substances they are not designed to deal with. When we eat food from mass-producing, non-local, non-organic suppliers, we risk ingesting pesticides, hormones, or other dangerous substances. Simply overloading our systems with an excess of food also creates a toxic imbalance. There are other toxins we may choose to take in recreationally, like drugs or cigarette smoke. Many of the medications we are prescribed to deal with our various ailments are in fact highly toxic. Even though they are effective in treating our acute symptoms, we need look no farther than all of the side effects—the tiny type on the back of the box, or the mandatory warnings spoken very quickly at the end of the TV ads—to know these medications have toxic potentials. We should still take these medications if we need them, but it is important to understand all the elements that create the high levels of toxicity our bodies are dealing with. Perhaps most importantly there are also emotional and psychological toxins that affect us: things such as stress, tension, anger, blame, fear, anxiety, negative thinking, and so on. The imbalance of our thoughts and emotions is most often the reason we cannot break the cycles of our toxic behaviors. Our bodies have a natural healing energy within us, but when overloaded with too much toxic behavior it cannot focus on reversing the disease process. It can only work keeping us to the status quo. Once we eliminate the toxic behavior, only then can our body's healing energies work on reversing the disease process rather than simply mitigating the damage.

Understanding Chronic Disease

Chronic disease is one of the hardest things for both patients and doctors to understand, and it's a problem we urgently need to grasp. Chronic diseases are now the leading cause of disability and death in the U.S., with seven of 10 deaths attributed to illnesses such as heart disease, cancer, and diabetes. One hundred and thirty-three million Americans have been diagnosed with at least one chronic disease, and more than one in 10 have three or more. On top of the tremendous cost in lives, chronic diseases account for 75 percent of the two trillion dollars spent each year on health care. On average, people with one chronic condition see three different physicians and fill seven prescriptions per year, while people with five or more chronic diseases make 12 physician visits and fill 50 prescriptions per year.

In Western society, chronic disease doesn't fit very well into our habitual way of thinking. We tend to think of disease in very black and white terms: either you have it or you don't. Unfortunately, this type of thinking limits our ability to understand its insidious nature. Chronic disease begins as an imbalance, or a distortion of energy flow. It is a state of being that is "out of sync" with natural laws. Initially, the toxicity is minimal and imperceptible. But if the pattern continues, slowly but surely the distorted energy flow will manifest as one of the familiar chronic disease states. Have you ever seen a rock formation in a cavern where water has dripped on the same spot over and over again? Each drip may seem insubstantial compared to the solidity of the rock beneath, but over time those drips will always win, eventually carving a deep pathway in the rock.

In the same way, we get high blood pressure a little at a time. It starts out quite early in life as an energy imbalance, with only minimal effects on our blood vessels. If the energy imbalance persists as we grow older, we lose those youthful reserves, and our blood vessels modify to accommodate the imbalance that our energy can no longer keep stabilized. It then seems we have suddenly developed a new disease state when, in fact, our inner healing energies have been dealing with the problem for a much longer time. We were just unaware of it. Chronic disease is the natural response to the toxic behaviors we have chosen for ourselves. It is a slow downward spiral. Because it is so subtle, however, it is often difficult to link the behaviors to the condition that ensues. If you doubt that our lifestyles play a central role in the onset of these diseases, you need look no further than the fact that other cultures with different lifestyles— such as the rural Chinese or the Maasai tribe in Africa—simply don't have heart disease or the other chronic conditions associated with Western society.

Chronic disease processes take a long time to manifest into their full-blown form. They remain under the radar for many years, especially if we are living a relatively active lifestyle. Coronary artery disease can start to develop in our early teens, which has been shown in autopsies on soldiers who were found to have narrowing of the arteries. Despite their military level of fitness combined with their youth, these young men were on their way to a heart attack. Poor dietary choices coupled with hereditary factors were already leaving their deadly mark.

There is an old Dutch proverb that says, "Sickness comes on horseback but departs on foot." The Chinese have a similar saying: "The appearance of a disease is swift as an arrow; its disappearance slow, like a thread." Such sentiments are true of many diseases, but when it comes to chronic disease, they could not be more wrong. Sometimes the symptoms may appear suddenly—like a heart attack or a diabetic shock—but the imbalance that led to these conditions has been building slowly and imperceptibly over a long period of time. Where the proverbs ring true is that it can take a long time for us to reverse these conditions. Chronic disease comes on foot and departs on foot, step by step. And just as we were the ones who created the path for it to arrive, we have to create the path for its departure.

The point is not to assign blame for your condition; it is to put the healing process in perspective. You can become empowered on your path to improve your health, but this can happen only if you are willing to understand and accept, without judgment, your own role in your current condition. If we can accept the fact that chronic disease results from an imbalance, and that it is an imbalance that, in large part, we created, then we can start to redress the balance. My hope is that when you truly understand why we get heart disease, the treatment will appear as nothing more than common sense. One of my favorite sayings is, "We don't beat heart disease; we come to terms with it."

CHAPTER 6

Heart Disease Demystified

"We all have an inner teacher, an inner guide, an inner voice that speaks very clearly but usually not very loudly. That information can be drowned out by the chatter of the mind and the pressure of day-to-day events. But if we quiet down the mind, we can begin to hear what we're not paying attention to. We can find out what's right for us."

—DEAN ORNISH

NOW THAT WE have redefined the concept of disease and have worked with the concepts of energy flow and balance, it is time to apply this new model to the physiological facts we know about heart disease. Understanding the mechanics of this condition will help you in your efforts to reverse or prevent this deadly killer.

Coronary artery disease is actually very simple. It is a wear-and-tear phenomenon that is due to repetitive injury. Imagine a busy road that is used every day by heavily-loaded trucks, cars, and buses in the heat of summer, the freezing cold of winter, and the heavy rains of fall and spring. Slowly but surely, the pavement will crack and erode, and if the traffic is not stopped once in a while to allow the damage to be repaired, the potholes will get so bad they can become dangerous, causing accidents and injury. In the same way, our arteries are subjected to repetitive injury that ultimately leads to cholesterol narrowings, or atheromatous plaques, which can, over time, lead to a heart attack. Plaque creates a disruption in blood flow by two different mechanisms. First, it narrows the lumen, or opening in the artery, and second, it causes the artery to act in a paradoxical manner by constricting when it should dilate. A normal artery's inner dimensions do not have physical narrowings and will dilate when the arterial wall senses an increase in blood flow to accommodate an increase in the demand for oxygen, such as when we are exercising or walking up stairs. If there is a significant narrowing, or stenosis, and the artery constricts, then blood flow is diminished. If the blood flow is ultimately diminished enough in a coronary artery (an artery that supplies blood flow to the heart), the heart muscle will become starved of oxygen, resulting in the symptom that we commonly refer to as "angina," or chest pain. This is why people with coronary heart disease can experience pain when they increase their activity level and during times of severe emotional stress. If these symptoms are brought on by exertion and that person then stops the activity and relaxes, the angina will go away. In this instance, there was not any damage done to the heart muscle; there was only a temporary disruption of blood flow.

If during exercise or a stressful situation one of these plaques ruptures, however, then a clot will form at the site of the rupture in an attempt to heal the artery. If this clot is large enough, it can completely cut off the blood flow to the heart muscle, causing damage to the heart. This is what is commonly referred to as a "heart attack." The sooner blood flow is restored, the less damage there will be to the heart. That is why heart attack patients need to get to the hospital as quickly as possible. If you were in the emergency room with chest pain and an electrocardiogram (ECG) showed you were having a heart attack, you would be rushed to the cardiac catheterization laboratory where an angiogram would take place to locate the blocked artery. After the blocked artery was identified, a wire would be guided through the clot, which would break it up and allow blood flow to be restored. Then an angioplasty (dilation of the artery with a balloon) would be performed, and most likely a stent (a device that helps to keep the artery open) would be inserted in order to prevent the ruptured plaque from closing down again, thus preventing another heart attack.

In the way I've just described it, coronary artery disease is the result of the accumulation of plaque within the walls of the arteries that supply the muscle of the heart with oxygen and nutrients. And while this is an accurate description of how we get heart disease, it is perhaps not the most useful one, because it doesn't tell the whole story. This limited definition brings to mind an image of something solid, hard, and literally calcified. It is hard to imagine something like that changing. This was the basis for the long-standing debate in the medical community on whether coronary artery disease, or any chronic condition, could be reversed. Now that you have the basic medical facts, let's look deeper into the underlying causes of coronary artery disease. In order to do this, I am going to ask you to think about it in a very different way.

Earlier in the book, I discussed energy and dis-ease. Heart disease can be reversed by restoring the "ease." Remember that everything in the universe has movement in it and there is a vibration in even the most solid objects, including rocks, metals, and, yes, coronary arteries. Let's look back at how heart disease develops. Long before the heart attack, the arteries were already in a dis-eased state, out of balance. It is important to note that before any physical abnormality in the blood vessel, the function of the blood vessel was already out of balance.

When we discuss coronary artery disease, the initial problem is defined by the medical term endothelial dysfunction. This is a fancy way of saying the arteries behave, or react, abnormally. Before there is even a little streak of fat on the wall of the artery, that blood vessel just simply misbehaves. How should an artery behave? As we mentioned before, when blood flows through a healthy coronary artery, the arterial wall will sense the pressure from the blood flow and respond by expanding, allowing more space for the larger volume of blood to flow smoothly. As the blood continues through, the healthy arterial wall will then respond with a soft contraction to restore the artery to its previous size. This expansion and contraction is called a pulsation.

A dis-eased artery will behave differently. In this case, when the blood travels down the dis-eased artery, instead of expanding to accept the blood, the artery will constrict, causing the blood flow to be distorted, or turbulent. To understand this, imagine putting your thumb over the edge of a garden hose with the water running. What happens when you do that? The water flows at an accelerated rate and sprays in all different directions. It is much harder to direct the stream of water to go where you want it to go.

The same thing happens in our arteries. When the dis-eased blood vessel senses the blood flowing through it, instead of dilating like it should, it constricts, causing the velocity of the blood flow to accelerate. And instead of the smooth, even flow in a healthy artery, this dysfunctional flow is erratic and strikes the arterial wall at awkward angles, creating areas of micro-trauma that, over time, will turn into lesions, or sites of inflammation. A lesion is the precursor of a cholesterol narrowing, or plaque.

The analogy I often use is that when you approach another person with a simple question, if everything is in balance, you will get a polite, informative, and truthful response. That would be "appropriate behavior." If there are mitigating circumstances in that person's life that create an imbalance, however, that same question asked exactly the same way might cause the person to be rude, refuse to answer, and even give misleading information. This kind of behavior is dysfunctional and inappropriate. Because the person was in a state of dis-ease, the response was dysfunctional. Our coronary arteries behave in much the same way.

Vascular Reconditioning

If we think of coronary artery disease in this way we can connect the dots to understand how yoga can reverse heart disease. When we practice yoga, we are in fact modifying our lifestyle in order to retrain our arteries to function normally. In this application, it is what I call a "vascular reconditioning" program. Thankfully, this vascular reconditioning can occur even in an artery that is 95 percent narrowed. In fact, once we begin to make the necessary changes in life, this can happen almost immediately. How do I know? It was one of the many breakthrough findings of Dr. Ornish's Lifestyle Heart Trial.

Besides the core revelation that yoga can reverse heart disease, to me one of the key findings of the Lifestyle Heart Trial is that minor reductions in the narrowing of the arteries can have major effects on the frequency, duration, and severity of the symptoms. It is important to slow down and focus on the information that I am going to share with you, because I think it is the most defining aspect of the study.

In Dr. Ornish's study, when angiograms were conducted on the yoga group after one year, it wasn't as if arterial narrowings of 90 percent were reduced to zero, or even 10 percent. Instead, the average reduction in the yoga group was from a narrowing of 40 percent to 37.8 percent. By contrast, in the usual care group, the narrowings increased from 42.7 percent to 46.1 percent.

As a cardiologist who has been doing catheterizations for more than 20 years, I can say most cardiologists looking at these results would not even be able to discern such a small degree of improvement or worsening of the narrowings with the naked eye. In fact, in order for the study to work, the angiograms were sent all over the country and readers were required to use a computer model to interpret the studies for accuracy and to prevent personal bias.

Given that the percentages were so small, what makes the results of this study so significant? For that, we need to consider that the frequency, or number of times, the participants had angina. In the yoga group, the number of angina events was reduced by a dramatic 91 percent, with a 42 percent reduction in the duration of the angina, and a 28 percent reduction in the severity of the angina. Comparatively, the usual care patients had a 165 percent increase in frequency of angina, a 95 percent increase in the duration of angina, and a 39 percent rise in the severity of angina.

The question I want you to consider is: If there were only a few percentage points difference on an angiogram, why was there such a dramatic improvement in symptoms? How can a minimal anatomic change result in such dramatic clinical results? I believe it is due to the vascular reconditioning that I referenced above. The yoga helped normalize the endothelial function in such a way that people who used to get chest pain walking halfway up a flight of stairs were now able to scale the stairs without any discomfort. The artery changed its behavior and acted differently.

Creating a Strong Foundation for Health

How does yoga do this? The answer comes back to energy— vibrational energy—and the rhythmic nature of that energy as it courses through our being and the arteries of our hearts. Let me explain.

The normal artery has three layers. There is an outer connective tissue layer called the adventitia; a middle muscular layer called the media, which influences the tone of the artery; and finally, the lining of the artery called the intima, or the endothelium. For years, the endothelium, which is only a single cell-layer thick, was thought to be inert, serving only to provide a barrier between the blood flow and the artery. It turns out, however, that the endothelium is the most important player in the evolution of coronary artery disease. This seemingly inert barrier is actually quite alive and is constantly secreting chemicals into the bloodstream that act locally on that segment of the coronary artery. When the artery is healthy, it secretes one set of chemicals that cause it to respond normally. When it is in dis-ease, it secretes another set of chemicals that result in endothelial dysfunction. So, in effect, what we are doing when we modify the behavior of our arteries is changing the chemicals that are secreted by the linings of our blood vessels. That is why we can get such a dramatic improvement in symptomatology with such a small improvement anatomically.

The results, as I have seen in my own patients, are incredible. I first met my patient, Sam, about 15 years ago. At the age of 45, he had all the classic symptoms of coronary artery disease. His stress test was abnormal, and he was sent to me for an evaluation and possible cardiac catheterization. After our initial workup, we discussed his options. I reviewed with him the data on reversing heart disease with yoga. We agreed to treat his disease process with a blended approach that included dietary modification, cardiac rehab, medical therapy, and a yoga-based cardiac wellness program. Within only a few weeks his chest pain was gone and one year later his stress test was completely normal. In fact, he was very competitive about exercise. Sam reversed his disease process, never had a cardiac catheterization, and never had a stent. What's more, over time, we reduced his medicine significantly, and he felt great. He stopped seeing me many years ago because he no longer required a cardiologist.

Remember the example I gave of how a person will sometimes respond rudely to a perfectly reasonable question because there are so many other things going on in his life? Imagine all of those issues get sorted out and that person is not only happy, but balanced, or in a state of ease. This time, when a question is asked, it gets the appropriate attention and response. The dysfunctional response had nothing to do with the question; it was due to pre-existing conditions. I often ask, if a building is constructed with a shaky foundation and wind comes by and knocks the building down, was it the wind or the foundation? When we treat the underlying cause and restore a strong foundation, we are able to respond appropriately on every level.

Healthful Evolutions affects vascular reconditioning by addressing the underlying cause. When the sink is overflowing, do we want merely to mop the floor while the water continues to run, or do we want to turn off the water? It seems like a silly question, but unless we understand the dynamics of the disease process, we can unknowingly be working against ourselves, rendering our best efforts, and those of our doctors, ineffective. Understanding the disease process allows you to take meaningful action to affect your own health at a much deeper level. You might still need medically-trained professionals to help you choose the right treatments for specific ailments, but you will already be creating the environment in which those treatments have the best chance of working, providing not only temporary relief from symptoms but lasting improvements in your health and quality of life.

PART 3

A PLAN FOR HEALTHY LIVING

CHAPTER 7

Learning to Breathe

"For breath is life, and if you breathe well you will live long on Earth."

—SANSKRIT PROVERB

HOW WE BREATHE determines how we experience the world. The breath nutrifies, detoxifies, affects every cell in our bodies, thereby governing how we feel, age, and deal with illness. The breath is literally everything. It's said that you don't know what you have until it's gone. When it comes to the breath we don't even know it is there, until it's not, and then we panic because we've never been taught how to breathe. In this chapter, we will learn why we breathe the way we do and the unintended consequences that we can expect if we don't intervene. Then we will explore SitStandStroll, the revolutionary technique that I have developed over the last 20 years that will allow you to connect to the power of your breath.

One of my patients, Paul, was a pack-a-day smoker with high cholesterol and high blood pressure when he suffered a heart attack at age 70. After being treated in the hospital with a coronary stent, he was sent home on several new medications. To Paul's credit, he did quit smoking for good, but his commitment to diet and exercise left a lot to be desired. Four years later he developed incapacitating arthritis in his neck resulting in a loss of balance and severe numbness and weakness in his hands, which led to a major orthopedic surgery. During the recovery period, his blood pressure became very difficult to control, and Paul ultimately required five blood pressure medications. That was when he finally agreed to participate in my cardiac reversal program, making it clear that the only reason he would attend was to improve his balance.

Within a few years, Paul's medical program included only a baby aspirin, one blood pressure medication, and no cholesterol-lowering drugs. He did not have any recurrent heart problems, and his balance, which was significantly affected by the spinal cord compression, stabilized. What enabled him to almost completely eliminate his multiple medications, improve his prognosis, and feel better had nothing to do with a new super drug, a new stent, or a new surgery. He learned how to breathe!

Considering that the breath is the most important function in our lives, you may wonder why breathing isn't taught in gym class instead of jumping jacks. This hasn't always been the case. For millennia, traditional healing practices centered their teachings on the breath, recognizing it as the basis for physical, emotional, and spiritual well-being. Just like the current in a flowing river, your breath creates a force, and all forces have consequences; they are never neutral. There are two basic breathing patterns that I refer to as FaceBreathing and BodyBreathing. FaceBreathing is the dysfunctional default pattern of breathing that most of us do unconsciously. BodyBreathing is the foundation practice of SitStandStroll that is going to change your life, forever.

Observing the Breath

Your goal, right now, is to develop a sense of your breath. Standing upright, take in a slow deep breath and notice what is happening. Don't change anything about the way you are standing or breathing and don't concern yourself about whether or not what you are doing is correct. If you are like most people, your face and neck muscles are the first to engage as you simultaneously draw in your stomach, lift your diaphragm, and expand your chest. This is FaceBreathing.

As you FaceBreathe you will notice that your upper body becomes top heavy as you draw up into your chest with each in-breath. This is due to the force exerted by the flowing energy of the in-breath. Feel your center of gravity migrate from your lower body and belly into your chest and head, making your upper body even more top-heavy, breath, after breath, after breath.

Now look at your feet, without changing anything. You are probably standing with your feet splayed towards the 10 and two o'clock positions, your hips are forward, your butt is back, and your shoulders are forward. Again, don't try to change this, just observe. This is an important distinction because it calls attention to the additive effect of how you stand, affecting your posture. When you FaceBreathe, you are not only breathing up, you are actually breathing up and forward due to the force of the breath following your body alignment. Therefore, your breathing habits are not just about how you breathe; they are also about how you stand.

The Consequences of FaceBreathing

As with all chronic dis-ease states, the negative effects of FaceBreathing are not immediately apparent and take decades to manifest. This demonstration will help you appreciate the untoward consequences of FaceBreathing. Begin by standing up and then taking two or three deep FaceBreaths. To understand the difficulty you will experience when you get older, allow your shoulders to slouch in an exaggerated fashion while bending forward at your waistline and then take a few more FaceBreaths. Notice how your breath is restricted by your upper body as your chest physically gets in the way. Now, walk in place for a few steps and then add the "old age" element—releasing your shoulders and bending forward at the waistline—and experience, first hand, how it becomes increasingly more difficult to breathe and walk at the same time when you are hunched over. It saddens me when I see my elderly patients struggle down the hallway bent over their walkers and canes. Many cannot come to the office anymore because they are bedbound due to their deteriorating body structure. What is even more disturbing is that this suffering is preventable as our bodies fail in a very predictable fashion.

FaceBreathing is a chronic dis-ease with serious implications. The solution is the BodyBreath, which will not only help to mitigate the negative effects of FaceBreathing on our physical structure, but will also play a major role in the prevention and reversal of heart disease.

Breathe Like a Baby

As infants and toddlers we BodyBreathe instinctively, cultivating a healthy, grounding energy flow that allows us not only to stand, but to navigate on the earth without a second thought. The irony is that we start out BodyBreathing; FaceBreathing takes over later in life. Through observing and treating people of all ages, I have pinpointed when and why this transition occurs.

An infant in his first weeks of life is a helpless creature whose only job is to eat, sleep, poop, and pee. He doesn't breathe like a marine with his stomach in and his chest out; instead his whole body expands with each in-breath like a lizard on a rock. As he develops, becoming bigger and stronger—no longer content with lying in his bed enjoying twenty-four-hour room service—he wants to lift up his head to see what's going on in the world but can't because he hasn't the strength or coordination to do so. Intuitively he starts the process by squeezing the muscles in his legs, lower back, and torso, curling up his little back like a cobra in order to sneak a quick peek around the room and then flop back to the ground. Whew! Imagine the concentration and effort required to accomplish such a monumental feat. He doesn't stop there. He continues to practice (he doesn't have much else to do) and pretty soon can keep his head up with less and less effort. In time he learns to push himself up on his hands and eventually to crawl, propelling himself across the floor. Finally, he is standing and ready to take his first steps.

I remember how exciting it was when my daughter was taking her first steps. We would go to a nearby park, which she loved because there were always lots of dogs. She would pull herself up, step one, step two, eyes focused on her feet, and then she would see a dog. Bam! She would lose her concentration and fall on her butt. Luckily, she thought this was funny.

Over time, her gait improved, and the dogs became a help rather than a hindrance. She would stand up, see a dog in the distance, put her head down, and motor her way over there. She still could not look up, however, because she hadn't yet mastered walking and thus needed to focus her attention on her feet to keep from falling, which was amusing because, more often than not, when she arrived at her destination the dog was gone. She would look around, find another dog, and start again. She did this over and over until walking became second nature, which meant she no longer needed to think about walking; she could just walk. To her delight, she found many more dogs and life was good. This is the moment that she, and all of us, unwittingly begins the transition from BodyBreathing to FaceBreathing, however.

When we no longer need to concentrate in order to remain upright and walk, we become FaceBreathers and spend the greater part of our lives unconsciously re-patterning our internal energy flows, allowing our center of gravity to migrate up and forward in our body structure, resulting in the top-heavy, old-age posture we would desperately like to avoid.

Why Does This Happen?

You may wonder, if we are born breathing in such a healthy way, why would we ever give it up? As with all chronic dis-ease states, the untoward manifestations of the dis-ease are not readily apparent to us. Because they don't appear in a significant way until many years later, the connection between the dis-ease entity and the cause is not immediately apparent. Even though we don't necessarily feel good when we eat poorly—other than, perhaps, the few minutes while we are actually eating the food—we don't feel bad enough, and continue on. Why would anyone ever start to smoke cigarettes or cigars? The body does everything it can to give us clues that we should stop; we cough, feel sick, get short of breath, smell bad, but we refuse to quit even when giving up smoking becomes a matter of life or death. This happens because we have cultivated internal energy flows I like to call HabitEnergy. HabitEnergies are practiced routines that we have integrated into our lives, for better or worse. Because they have been so deeply entrenched into our beings, to live any other way feels awkward, as if something is off or missing. This is why unhealthy HabitEnergies are so difficult to break. FaceBreathing is nothing more than another HabitEnergy. We learn it watching our parents, or in gym class when we are told to stand straight with our stomachs in and our chests out. Women confide that they are taught this is how a "lady" carries herself. Clearly, FaceBreathing has a cultural component, and understandably we conform to the norm. As infants and toddlers, we walk with intention, deeply focused on the present moment because we have to in order to keep from falling. When we master the movement and are no longer in fear of falling, however, our intention and attention shifts to other matters, and our inner energy flows adjust. Soon FaceBreathing feels normal and becomes our new HabitEnergy.

Establishing a New HabitEnergy

BodyBreathing is the foundation practice of SitStandStroll that will not only counteract the postural problems caused by FaceBreathing, but also set the stage for the prevention and reversal of coronary artery disease by establishing a new, healthful HabitEnergy.

EXERCISE

Begin standing, being careful not to use the muscles in your face and neck. Inhale while tightening the muscles around your ankles, your calves, and then your thighs, sequentially engaging the legs from your feet to your hips. Maintaining the engagement in your legs, tighten the muscles around your low back, your middle back, and then your upper back. You are now at the top of the in-breath and should feel the air flowing into your lungs through your mouth or nose. As you start your out-breath, imagine your breath flowing down your back, down your butt, thighs, calves, and feet into the floor. Believe it or not, that is the BodyBreath. Could it be that simple?

With BodyBreathing you will notice that your upper body becomes lighter with each in-breath. You are standing straighter, and you are doing a diaphragmatic breath, which is the most powerful relaxation response in your body. Above all, you are practicing a yoga-based activity by integrating your mind, your body, and your breath in a single action, which has been shown to lower cholesterol, lower blood pressure, reverse heart disease, and reduce stress, as well as provide many other numerous benefits.

All of this is happening because you are breathing in a completely different way. Feel your jaw relax as your face and neck muscles finally take a break. You can stop grinding your teeth anytime you want. As you practice, your mind and body do their best to convince you to use your facial muscles to initiate the breath; this sensation in your facial muscles is simply a HabitEnergy that does not want to be denied. As you continue to practice BodyBreathing, the urge to FaceBreathe will wane, and a new HabitEnergy rooted in the BodyBreath will take over. Most importantly, you are engaging your body the same way an infant does when he takes his first look around the room. You are breathing like a baby.

A BodyBreath is a much deeper breath than the FaceBreath. With FaceBreathing, the face and neck muscles, shoulders, and maybe the upper torso are utilized in addition to drawing the diaphragm up into the chest, which ultimately serves to decrease the volume of air flowing into the lungs. With BodyBreathing, the process of breathing begins in the feet and ankles and then works its way sequentially up the legs and spine, causing the diaphragm to draw down towards the feet, which increases the volume of air flowing into the lungs.

A major factor that distinguishes BodyBreathing from FaceBreathing is the out-breath, or exhalation. The first thing that most people do when they think of taking a breath is to inhale. In order to experience the deepest breath possible, however, one must exhale first. If you have a glass of water and it is a quarter empty, you can refill it only 25 percent, no matter how much water you pour in. If you empty the glass completely, however, you can fill it 100 percent. When you BodyBreathe, you begin with the out-breath and you extend it all the way down to your feet. Now initiate the in-breath with the "glass" 100 percent empty, filling it from the bottom up.

Integrating and Grounding

EXERCISE

While standing, slowly BodyBreathe. After a fewseconds, at the beginning of an out-breath, feel the flow of energy down your spine, down your thighs, calves, and ankles as it travels to the floor. As this occurs you will notice your legs tightening, or integrating. They feel stronger, more compact. Hold on to this tightness in your legs as you begin your next in-breath at your ankles. This will impart an exaggerated grounding sensation as your legs draw even more firmly into the floor. It is important to note that there is a direct correlation with how integrated the body is and the depth of your out-breath, which will in turn correlate with the magnitude of the in-breath.

Begin the next in-breath with the legs firmly engaged and then BodyBreathe up the legs and spine. On the out-breath, continue the engagement in the legs as the energy travels down the body into the feet. Feel the additional "squeeze" and notice how much more stable your legs become. Don't let go! BodyBreathe again and realize that this is not only making the out-breath deeper; it allows more room for a fuller in-breath and, increasingly, creates a sense of lightening of your upper body at the same time.

My patients will often ask me if they should relax their leg muscles on the in-breath or the out-breath because it almost seems unnatural not to take a break. The reality is that we want them to be engaged all of the time, and this exercise highlights the importance of the principle engagement. When a muscle is constantly engaged we say that it is toned even though we are not lifting weights. When we, as human beings, are 100 percent engaged in what we are doing, life is better.

Rooting

A friend of mine was building a house on a lakeshore. Specialized support beams, or pylons, were planted deep into the earth to support the structure because the land was so mushy. If the pylons were not deep enough, the house would sink. This helped me understand that we could not simply rest our own feet on the earth; instead, we need to root our own pylons deep, deep into the earth as we navigate the mushy foundations in our own lives.

EXERCISE

While standing, guide the out-breath down your spine and legs and then extend the out-breath through your feet and into the floor, rooting the breath five, 10, 15, 20 feet, deep, deep into the earth. Observe the effect on your body. Notice how the deeper you root, the more you engage, or integrate, your lower body. Notice, once again, that the more you integrate, the lighter your upper body becomes. Your legs become infinitely more stable, and the next in-breath begins spontaneously.

EXERCISE

Now that we know how to root, hold that engagement in your legs and begin another BodyBreath. The grounding experience continues to deepen and your upper body lightens even more. Let's add another layer to this concept of integration. At the end of the next out-breath, root as previously described, but this time actively push your feet and legs into the floor as you begin the sequential engagement up your legs. Relax the muscles in your face and neck; let the rest of your body do the work of breathing. Notice the difference in the quality of the in-breath now that you have deeply rooted your legs into the earth, just as my friend did with the pylons of his lake house.

A Quick Review

This is a good time to review what we have learned and what our goals are. FaceBreathing is a chronic dis-ease. It is the default, dysfunctional breathing pattern with side effects that are so subtle we never know that anything is amiss but that, nevertheless, have a profound long-term effect on our lives. FaceBreathing's un-grounding energy flow can lead to increased anxiety, high cortisol levels, hypertension, high cholesterol, diabetes, coronary artery disease, as well as the slumped over posture that we associate with old age. We naturally BodyBreathe as infants and toddlers, but when we no longer have to intentionally ground our feet into the earth to walk we began the transition from BodyBreathing to FaceBreathing.

BodyBreathing is the cornerstone practice of SitStandStroll and is the solution to FaceBreathing. The BodyBreath is a grounding breath comprised of the in-breath and the out-breath. We begin with the out-breath, emptying the "glass." The in-breath grounds our legs and feet into the earth and creates lightness in our upper body. At no time during the process are we using our face, neck, or shoulders to help with the BodyBreath! Appreciate how the body is able to generate enough suction to draw the air from the atmosphere into the lungs without the aid of the head and neck. Also notice how the face still wants to "do the job" of breathing. This sensation that you are "breathing wrong" is due to a HabitEnergy you have cultivated over the previous decades.

Take time to feel what is happening inside of you as you begin to make the transition from FaceBreathing to BodyBreathing. Most people feel they have to FaceBreathe in order to receive enough oxygen into their bloodstream even though with a BodyBreath they have actually taken a deeper breath. There is always resistance with change, both internal and external. HabitEnergies are practiced routines that create muscle, or metabolic, memory within our bodies that needs to be modified.

SitStandStroll can help you modify your HabitEnergy so that it is in line with the universal laws of nature. Dis-eased coronary arteries constrict rather than dilate when blood flows through them. Our goal is to change the HabitEnergy of the lining of the arteries, the endothelium, so they dilate when blood flows through. It's that simple. The BodyBreath is directly connected to the endothelium of your coronary arteries!

You are now choosing your destiny. Our ultimate goal is to improve our lives. We do that by modifying our HabitEnergies. We are creating a new HabitEnergy with the BodyBreath as we pulsate the energy up and down our spines. In turn we will become accustomed to a deep, full BodyBreath rather than the shallow FaceBreath that we have been doing for most of our lives. This pulsing energy flow will help to create other more healthful HabitEnergies, including in the arteries of our heart as you are now reversing heart dis-ease and cultivating the ease in your blood vessels that your body craves.

Levitating On the Earth

In order to be fully engaged we must ground ourselves, both physically and mentally. Grounding is an action that anchors our lower bodies into the floor by the sequential engagement of legs and thighs. As you execute this action, your upper body will feel lighter with each and every breath.

EXERCISE

At the end on your next out-breath, tighten your ankles, then your calves, and now your thighs. Stop. Did you feel it? Your feet and legs are pushing into the floor, and your upper body is floating up. Why? Because you have grounded your body. Amazing! Now, extend this engagement up your spine and feel it lengthen. You have just begun the process of reversing back dis-ease by creating space between the vertebrae in your spine. Continue to practice this grounding exercise and feel your upper body become lighter and lighter every day, the same way it was becoming heavier and heavier before you knew what was happening.

A Deeper Breath

As you use your body and breath to pulsate the energy up and down your spine, you also increase energy flows in all of the cells in your body due to the more efficient exchange of oxygen and carbon dioxide. This pulsation is connected to everything. It calms the nervous system, improves digestion, and improves the health of the arteries in your heart.

When we breathe, we are simply moving energy with a nutrifying in-breath and detoxifying out-breath. The body is nothing more than an energy pump. The more efficient we are in this "energy transfer," the better our lives; it's that simple. I find it funny how our lives are so backwards. We do everything to make our lives more complicated when we crave simplicity. We look outward for answers when the solution is found within. The breath is the key to everything, and how we experience it is how we experience life.

This is a great moment as we start to celebrate one of many "firsts." We become very excited for our children's firsts—the first time they see snow, swim in the ocean, fly on an airplane, walk, and so on.

Take part in the same joy that you have been saving for others and allow some for yourself. We all possess unlimited joy, and you will get better at accessing it as you practice (another new HabitEnergy). Cultivate the kind of awareness, concentration, and engagement in your body and being that you left behind before breathing, standing, and walking became second nature to you.

Gravity Can Be Your Friend

People view gravity as a detrimental force, especially when it comes to aging. It accelerates our bad posture and causes our skin to sag. Indeed, gravity may be the most pervasive natural force our bodies have to deal with. As we explore how our bodies interact with gravity, the beneficial effects of BodyBreathing and grounding are immediately apparent. Gravity is necessary for our survival and can actually aid us in an anti-aging process as we align with the laws of nature.

Gravity has a flow and is always directed towards the center of the earth. Like everything else in nature, gravity is neither good nor bad. How it affects us depends on how we relate to it. While we cannot alter the energy flow of gravity, we can alter the energy flows within our own bodies, the most powerful of which is the breath. As we have seen, how we stand and how we breathe determines the internal energy flows in our bodies. The big problem is how our bodies respond when these two forces meet. Where they meet, or interface, opportunity exists.

I think that we can all agree that our body structure, or the force of our breath, will never overwhelm the force of gravity. We are decidedly disadvantaged in this balancing act. So, our goal is to come to terms with gravity and how we can relate to it. If our physical structure and energy flow are compromised, we will falter just like Charlie Brown's anemic Christmas tree that breaks down when a single ornament is hung on it. Adding more stress (gravity) to an already compromised system (our failing body structure) can only lead to disaster. With BodyBreathing and grounding we are able to redirect the added stress of gravity in such a way that it actually becomes an anti-aging force.

Think back to the differences in our body alignment when we compared FaceBreathing and BodyBreathing. Breathing with your face raises you up and tips you forward. The force of gravity causes your misaligned head and top-heavy upper body to weaken as they are suspended in space without proper support. In time, the force of gravity will cause this weakened, top-heavy body to bend severely, or even break. It is a simple matter of physics.

To compare, let's go back to the BodyBreathing technique where the practice relies on sequential engagement of the body from feet to head on the in-breath, and then from head to feet on the out-breath. When we are engaged and aligned, instead of gravity pushing the body forward and down, our body's rising internal energy behaves like an arrow cutting through gravity, streaming towards the sky. This occurs because the force of gravity is deflected and flows down the sides of our aligned structures, hugging its edges, and when we initiate the next in-breath, the grounding action draws that same energy up through our core. This weightlessness and expansion is a natural property of energy. Now gravity is working for us, not because we have overwhelmed it, but because we have taken the time to understand it and redefine our relationship with the universal laws of nature.

Advanced Exercises

1. ADVANCED GROUNDING

With your next out-breath, root deeply into the earth. Simply keep your legs and body firmly engaged and actively push your feet and legs into the floor without repeating the active sequential engagement of the muscles up the legs and spine. Notice that the breath flows in on its own through this process of rooting. All of a sudden, the in-breath seems to occur effortlessly.

As we root, the legs, ankles, calves, and thighs engage spontaneously, and the grounding energy flow expands and lightens the upper body. On the next out-breath, follow the rooting energy flow, deep, deep, deep into the earth, even deeper than before. Feel how the deeper you go, the harder your legs work. On your next in-breath, with no face muscle nor active sequential engagement, accentuate the rooting by guiding the breath deeper and deeper into the earth. Feel your legs engage, and actively push your feet and your legs into the earth. Now, simply lift your shoulders up towards your ears, which will lengthen your torso and spine. Make sure there isn't any clenching in your shoulders, neck, or face, and revel in the sequential opening and lightness that is ascending up your body. Wow!

2. EMPTY THE GLASS

At the top of the in-breath, begin the out-breath and, as it descends down the spine, curl your body forward expelling as much of your breath as possible, like you are wringing all of the water out of a sponge. Your torso will bend forward like the letter "C." At the end of the out-breath, with your body curled in as tight as you can, push your feet and legs into the floor and simultaneously straighten your body, creating a much bigger in-breath. Repeat the process several times and intentionally pulsate the breath, or energy, in and out of your body as if you are an energy pump (which is actually what you are). I liken the action to that of a jellyfish as it undulates through the water, drawing and expelling the water through its body to create movement.

By creating a deeper out-breath, we are able to deepen the in-breath. Recall our glass of water from earlier. If it is one quarter empty, we can only fill it 25 percent no matter how much water we have. If we empty the glass 100 percent, however, we can fill it with more water.

Let's try again. On your next out-breath, empty the glass all of the way down and root your energy deep, deep into the earth. Now, with your body fully integrated and engaged, open it up and let the air flow in as you push your feet into the floor and simultaneously straighten out your upper body. Feel how your body fills, or expands, on the in-breath and then, on the next out-breath, feel the integration as you BodyBreathe down through the floor and start the process over and over again.

Mastering the BodyBreath

BodyBreathing may be the most important foundational practice of a healthy lifestyle. There is nothing more important to the body than the breath. It is the first thing that we do when we are born and the last thing that we do before we die. It is the difference between life and death. When you learn to breathe in this way, it will change your life. Savor each breath because, as we have learned, it will ground you emotionally and physically and is the key to everything.

Don't worry if you find these exercises difficult to master. It may take a little while to get the hang of it, or it may take just a minute. It's like learning how to ride a bicycle. Sometimes it is challenging at first, but once you know how, you never forget. As you continue with the practice it will get easier. Be patient. In the beginning, you will notice the shift in the directionality and flow of your breath. When you are able to experience this shift, you will be able to sense, and then balance, the breath against the force of gravity. As you will see in the next chapter, you can apply this technique throughout your day, and soon it will become second nature.

This is a subtle practice and takes time. It works on many different levels. When we first begin to practice a healthy lifestyle that includes diet, exercise, and SitStandStroll, we cultivate an environment for our arteries to respond normally. We cannot expect to reverse decades of abuse overnight; the arteries will begin to respond normally, however, as we have identified an unhealthy energy flow and replaced it with a new, healthy HabitEnergy.

CHAPTER 8

Practicing SitStandStroll™ Yoga

"Yoga takes you into the present moment, the only place where life exists."

"Constant practice alone is the secret of success."
—HATHA YOGA PRADIPIKA

THE YOGA SUTRAS, written by Patanjali around 400 CE, espouses the science of yoga that had been evolving for several millennia. In its original form, the practice of yoga may at first seem out of reach for most of us; its teachings continue to be relevant today, however, as we enter this new age in health care. For instance, did you know that people who meditate regularly use the medical system 70 percent less than those who don't? Also, a Mutual of Omaha study on the effects of Dr. Ornish's cardiac reversal program demonstrated a savings of $200 for every $1 spent on the cost of the program. In fact, lifestyle practices—like yoga and meditation—that would have been routinely dismissed as quackery or placebo medicine in the past are garnering more attention today in an effort to reduce health care costs and improve the quality of life.

SitStandStroll is a powerful yoga practice that honors and takes advantage of all that yoga has to offer. Most people think of yoga as a form of physical exercise, but traditional yoga is all encompassing, and, as eluded to above, it is a science. If you take the time to read one of the many versions of the Yoga Sutras, you will be more than surprised. It made me realize that there is the external universe with which we are all acquainted—filled with planets, stars, galaxies, and black holes—and then there is an inner universe we discover only when we close our eyes and look within. The irony is that the inner universe mirrors the outer universe, so we can learn what we need to know through a process of deep introspection. It was Patanjali who organized the yogic method so others could learn how to experience this inner universe themselves.

Once we understand that there is healing energy pulsing through our bodies and beings constantly, then we know the next step is to learn how to access it as fully as possible. SitStandStroll helps connect us with that healing energy. As one of the great yoga masters, B.K.S Iyengar, explained, "Yoga, an ancient but perfect science, deals with the evolution of humanity. This evolution includes all aspects of one's being, from bodily health to self-realization. Yoga means union—the union of body with consciousness and consciousness with the soul. Yoga cultivates the ways of maintaining a balanced attitude in day-to-day life and endows skill in the performance of one's actions." Simply stated, yoga encompasses literally everything that we do: how we eat, think, act, exercise ... you name it. This may seem dramatic, but its relevance cannot be overstated; because we now know that everything we do is important, we also know that nothing is irrelevant. Yogic philosophy actually makes it easier for us understand and integrate the causes and consequences of our actions to health and well-being. As we review our health goals, we internalize the fact that everything we do is important. From an energy standpoint, our mission is to modify our bodies' reactivity—our HabitEnergies—in relation to the environment in which we live. By living consciously and with awareness, a vascular reconditioning process takes place, resulting in the prevention and reversal of heart disease. This is accomplished because we have aligned with the universal laws of nature, and, as suggested by B.K.S. Iyengar, this is a full-time job that requires paying attention to every aspect of our lives and much more than an hour a week in a yoga studio to make it happen.

Yoga is a lifestyle. Above all, yoga is about awareness and engagement. It is about making conscious choices and cultivating new HabitEnergies through practice. Here's an example that may not sound like yoga in the usual sense. I am a strong advocate of home blood-pressure monitoring, and I encourage all my patients to record their blood pressure daily because it aids me in the treatment of their hypertension and also makes them a partner in their own healing process. Although they may not know it, these patients are in fact practicing yoga as they become more aware of and engaged with their health treatment. Often, when they first start taking their blood pressure, they will not like the results; their blood pressure reading will be too high. When they see these readings, however, they stop, relax, take a few deep breaths, and then retake their blood pressure, hoping for a better result, which they usually will get. This is often their first experience with mind-body medicine. After a while, they will get used to taking their blood pressure every day, and it will seem odd to them if they don't (another example of a new HabitEnergy). When they record their weight with their blood pressure, they see firsthand how their blood pressure responds to fluctuations in their weight, as well as to what they are eating and whether or not they are exercising. It is amazing to see how happy people become when they finally get their blood pressure under control, especially if it has been a long-standing problem. Some patients even share that they can tell what their blood pressure will be before they take it, based on how they feel.

SitStandStroll is an authentic yoga-based healing program because it continuously reminds you to bring your awareness to your breath. What I am most proud of is that this method is accessible to anyone no matter how young or old they are. Many of my patients who benefit most are in their 70s, 80s, and 90s because they are in the most pain and distress and are willing to work the hardest. So, even if you are well into your golden years, it's not too late to begin.

This is the good stuff! You are acquiring the tools to make the transformative changes in your body structure that you never thought possible. You are now working in a completely different way—with an energy model. Understanding body alignment is vital, and there are a lot of details that will seem complex upon first reading but will become easier to understand as we go. Don't despair: soon you will get the "feel" of it, and then it will become second nature—so much so that you will wonder how you survived so long without it.

Remember, perfection is not the goal. If you are seeking "perfect," you will fail miserably. Perfection does not exist. You do not need to be in perfect alignment in order to reap the benefits of SitStandStroll, but having an ideal in mind will give us an idea of what we need to do in order to improve things. The reality is we are always in a transition process because our bodies, as well as our life situations, are always changing. We are either getting better or we are getting worse, and as we cultivate more awareness WE get to make the choice about which direction we want to go.

Yoga—Myths and Misunderstandings

Myth: Yoga is an exercise program.

Truth: The practice of yoga involves everything we do. When people ask me what is important, I tell them everything is important: what we eat, what we do, how we exercise, what we think, everything. That is why yoga is so powerful.

Hatha yoga is one aspect of the practice. Hatha is a term that we traditionally use to describe the asana practice, or the familiar poses and postures we associate with yoga. Realize that this is only part of the practice of yoga. You do not need to twist yourself into a pretzel in order to benefit. However, there is indeed a physical component to the practice. Don't let this intimidate you.

Myth: You need to be physically flexible to practice yoga.

Truth: If you were able to connect with the BodyBreathing exercise we reviewed earlier, then you are already doing yoga. When I first started practicing yoga, I was as stiff as a board. My teacher John Friend explained that flexibility is not about how far we can stretch our muscles; it is actually a combination of alignment and strength. This will become clear as you progress in the program. Let me assure you that, in time, you will become more flexible than you ever thought possible.

Myth: You can't hurt yourself doing yoga.

Truth: You can injure yourself doing yoga, which is why you want to be very careful as to how you go about it. A huge revelation for me came in a very unexpected fashion. Like so many others, I thought that being healthy had everything to with being flexible. When I discovered hatha yoga, I thought, "This is it!" My goal was to be able to palm the floor when doing a forward bend, and I worked hard at it. Then, one day, I severely injured my knee during a yoga class. While I was in an awkward yoga pose, the teacher's instruction was, "Perhaps this is the day that you straighten your knee." When I did straighten my knee, I can't tell you how happy I was. What I didn't realize was that the "ca-chunk" sensation in my knee meant that I had just torn some cartilage! Stranger still, because I was so happy that I could finally straighten my knee in this pose, I kept doing it because I thought that I was succeeding at doing yoga. It wasn't until 10 or so days later, when my knee filled up with fluid, that I realized something was wrong.

I concede that this "just do it" approach may work for some people, especially if they are young and gifted with a lot of natural flexibility. More likely, however, this approach will lead to undesirable consequences such as my own. Note that I was in my 30s when I injured my knee and in what most people would describe as excellent shape, working out at least five days a week.

SitStandStroll

Before we begin, let's review. Our immediate goal is to learn how to alter the energy flows and HabitEnergies in our minds and bodies, which will in turn recondition our vasculature in order to prevent and reverse heart disease. We develop coronary artery disease because the unhealthy energy flows in our bodies cause our blood vessels to act abnormally. SitStandStroll helps transform this dysfunctional energy flow into a healthy flow. This transformational healing process begins by working with the energy flow that is most easily accessible to us: our breath.

SitStandStroll is a foundational practice that can benefit anyone: from the absolute beginner to the experienced practitioner. It is well suited for those of us who are at risk for injury, which includes essentially everybody. Being physically fit matters little when practicing yoga. I have had the unique opportunity to work with the senior population, as most of the participants in my Monday class are in their 70s and 80s, with a growing number in their 90s. Because SitStandStroll teaches you how to work your body safely, you will be able to attend any yoga class and reduce your risk of injury because you will have a greater awareness of what is right for your body and what isn't.

In the following pages, I share detailed instructions for each part of the SitStandStroll practice. I cannot emphasize this enough: if you do not try the practice, it will not make sense to you. Sometimes people like to read through it first to get an idea of where it is going, but if all you do is read it, you will not be able to benefit. As we begin, be patient with yourself as this may come easy for you or it may take a little time. I am fond of celebrating the transition periods of my life, particularly when it comes to mastering a life-changing skill. Sometimes it is good to try hard, and sometimes it is good to try easy. As you proceed, remind yourself that you don't have to have the "volume" cranked up all of the time. So please smile and enjoy yourself during the process; that may be the most meaningful yoga practice of all.

This is a cumulative practice, meaning that it builds on itself. There are a lot of similarities within each section. The Sit will teach you the Stand, which will teach you the Stroll, which will teach you the Stand, and so on. If, for whatever reason, some aspect of the practice doesn't make sense in one position, it will become clear in another. Relax. You haven't missed anything. Once you get the basics down, you will be doing this for the rest of your life.

SitStandStroll is effective and powerful because you can do it all day long. It pushes us to be totally engaged in the three things we are doing almost the entire day: sitting, standing, and strolling. People ask me whether they need to think about what they are doing all day. My usual response is that you are always thinking about something anyway, so why shouldn't it be something beneficial to you, like your overall health and well-being?

Stand

I call this practice SitStandStroll, but in fact I am going to teach it to you in a different order. We will start with the Stand component of the practice, the foundational pose of hatha yoga, called Tadasana, or Mountain Pose. Tadasana is often referred to as the most important pose in yoga because it is the one upon which all other poses are built. This will become clear in time, especially as you start working with more advanced poses and reflect on Stand as a reference point for body alignment.

Just as BodyBreathing is the foundational practice, Stand is the foundational pose. Now we are going to refine the BodyBreathing technique with alignment while in Stand. We'll begin with the feet. As in BodyBreathing, the first action is to ground our feet into the floor: how they are positioned is important. Begin by positioning your feet directly underneath your hips, so they are parallel to each other and about four to six inches apart. In order to make the feet parallel (because the shape of the feet are so irregular) draw an imaginary line from the middle your ankles to the bottom of the second toe (next to the big toe) and position these lines parallel to each other. Sometimes people will use some eyeliner or a washable marker as an aid. You may feel like you are standing pigeon-toed, but that's because we usually stand with our feet splayed. (This is another example of HabitEnergy when we become aware that a more healthful way of standing actually feels awkward, and our first instinct is to change our feet back to the more comfortable previous position even though it is less beneficial to our health and well-being.)

Let's play with this a little more. Without letting your heels leave the floor, balance your weight between your toes and your heels. Press the mounds of the big toes (the balls of your big toes) on each foot firmly into the floor and feel how this action draws your shins together. Put enough effort into this action so that the outside edges of your feet lift off the floor. Maintaining this action, allow your heels to sink into the floor and then draw the top of your ankles towards your heels. Notice how this causes your toes to spread and lift off the floor as you continue to press the mounds of the big toes into the floor. As you hold this engagement in your feet, draw the energy in your calf muscles up from the ankles towards the back of your knees and forward, strong enough so that they are pressing on the back of the shins and creating a soft bend, or micro-bend, in the knee (this protects the knee). This may take more effort than you are used to.

Next, locate the upper, inner aspects of your thighs (at your groin) and move them back like you are trying to moon the person behind you. In other words, really stick your butt back! Notice you have actively shifted your legs onto the back plane of your body. It should feel as if you are bending, or bowing forward, from your hips, not your waist. At this point, there may be a somewhat intense curve in your low back. Don't worry, because this is easily taken care of by drawing your belly button in towards your spine and curling your tailbone under. As you do this, the intense sensation in your lower back should go away. Does it feel weird yet? Please be patient; this will all be worth it.

If you haven't taken a break yet, this might be a good time to stop and shake your legs out. When you are ready, turn back the page and repeat the practice of engaging your lower body. Once your lower body is aligned, gently shrug your shoulders up towards your ear, move your upper arms to your backbody, and feel your shoulder blades on your back. Now BodyBreathe. Engage all the way from your feet to your upper back and then reverse the engagement all the way down your spine towards your feet on the out-breath. What do you feel? Hopefully, you feel a sequential engagement of your body from your feet to the base of your skull that should simultaneously create an in-breath and the sequential engagement in the opposite direction as you simultaneously create an out-breath. Try to make the sequential tightening of your muscles as smooth as possible as you pulsate the awareness up and down your spine; the in-breath on the way up and the out-breath on the way down. Leave the work of breathing to your body. Notice the HabitEnergy that you have cultivated over the years from FaceBreathing. Feel how, when you BodyBreathe, your face wants to be involved in the process. On your next in-breath, do everything you can to keep your face from participating. This is harder than you think.

As I stated above, SitStandStroll relies on continuous engagement, which also includes awareness. What is confusing for us Westerners is that we think that we have to be perfect. When we become aware of what we perceive as a bad HabitEnergy, many feel that this needs to resolve immediately. This is not the case. Allow yourself time to feel the sensations in a nonjudgmental fashion so that you not only feel comfortable with the existing HabitEnergy, you are comfortable as you transition to a new, more healthful HabitEnergy.

We are going to go over the process again, with more detail. It is your choice whether to proceed or continue to work on what we have already done. My advice is to plow through to the end and then start back at the beginning. Again, you do not have to master everything at once; I would feel very good if you picked up even five percent this first time through. There is no need to panic, as proficiency will come in time with continued practice. Please do not be critical of yourself as it will only slow down your progress.

Let's start again by first positioning your feet parallel, four to six inches apart from each other, and letting your heels sink into the floor while actively pressing the mounds of your big toes into the ground and drawing the base of your shins back towards the heels. Then create a drawing action in your calves from the heels through the Achilles tendon towards the back of the knees. Actively engage the calf muscles to create a micro-bend in the knee. Keeping the shins fully engaged, simply move your upper, inner thighs to the back plane of your body and widen your hips creating more space in your low back. Next, draw your navel to your spine and simultaneously draw your tailbone down, and then draw down from the back of your thighs towards the back of your knees, accentuating the micro-bend in your knees.

This next part is perhaps the most difficult to master. The kidney region is what I like to refer to as "no-man's land" because it was the most difficult area to bring awareness to. This is the area that occupies the space in your lower, middle back. Imagine drawing a line from your navel right through to your spine. Next, imagine another line that travels just below the lower border of your rib cage, where your diaphragm is located, to your spine. The area between these two lines is the kidney area. This is an area that requires special attention because it will, in time, become your secret weapon. Remember this area, as we will return to it in a moment.

Now we are going to work on our shoulders in a bit of a different way. Gently shrug your shoulders towards your ears, bring your upper arm bones towards your back body and then extend both arms straight out to either side so they are parallel to the floor with your palms facing forward. Spread out your fingers, bringing your attention to the pinky fingers on either hand. Draw energy primarily from your pinky finger to your wrist, forearm, and then your triceps (the lower aspect of your upper arms when they are extended out to either side), allowing that engagement to travel along the lower borders of your shoulder blades to the middle of your back. You should feel your shoulder blades flatten on your back as you draw the energy intensely from your hands, through your arms, and into the center of your back. Keeping the hands, arms, and shoulder blades fully engaged, send the energy from the center of your back out through your arms, hands, and to your fingertips. Allow this energy to pulsate from your fingertips into the center of your spine and then back out through your fingertips. Does this seem familiar? This is BodyBreathing for the upper arms! Same concept, same sequential engagement. See how it all builds on itself? Continue to pulse the energy in and out of your arms until they are slightly fatigued. You may feel a sensation like someone is pressing on the middle of your back. Now, draw in your upper abdomen (your solar plexus), let your chest rock forward slightly while you keep your shoulder blades fully engaged down your back, and drop your arms to your sides.

Once you have aligned the shoulders, gently tilt your skull forward at the point of your ear canal, or ear lobe. Imagine a line that starts on the upper lip, travels back through the palate, to the point of your ear lobes. With that in mind, reset your foundation. Sink your heels into the floor, actively draw up the calves strongly enough to micro-bend the knees, draw your navel to the spine, curl your tailbone down and under. Draw down from your pelvis to the back of the your thighs, to the back of the your knees, curl the your tailbone under again, and then draw your navel in again, but this time puff up the kidneys towards the lower aspect of the shoulder blades (the secret weapon). Now lift up through your torso, bend your elbows slightly, and draw your fully-engaged shoulder blades towards each other, integrating them with your entire neck up to the base of the skull, as if it were all one piece. Pause, settle, and re-engage.

Next, move your Adam's apple back towards the spine, creating a feeling of fullness in the back of your neck, as if you are breathing out of the back of your neck (like a fish breathes through its gills). Then shift the back of your neck and ears straight back, in one piece, and let the energy from the Adam's apple float back and up through the ear lobes and then up through the crown of the head. Let gravity sink the lower borders of the shoulder blades down the back as they are sweetly drawn together. Draw your navel towards your spine and then curl your tailbone down. Execute a fully engaged out-breath and then BodyBreathe with alignment.

Please take some time to notice how the alignment of Stand and the BodyBreathing work together. You can work on each separately, but when you combine the two, magic happens. My advice is to continue BodyBreathing at all times. When you have time to think about it, refine the practice with alignment. As you become more engaged with the practice, it will make a lot more sense to you. Also, notice that when you have some discomfort in your body, if you pause and align, frequently it is alleviated. This is a powerful principle that becomes more powerful with practice and patience. You are on your way to a better life.

Stroll

I would now like to shift gears and put what we have learned so far into motion as we Stroll, or walk. As you might expect, in order to re-learn how to walk, we begin in the Stand pose. So, let's resume BodyBreathing by starting with your ankles, calves, thighs, belly button, lower back, middle back, and upper back, followed by the sequential engagement down your back, butt, legs, and feet into the floor. Do this a few times so that you develop a flow. When you are ready, as your out-breath flows down your back, direct it into your right leg only. On the next in-breath, slowly engage the right ankle only, and let the engagement travel sequentially up the right leg and then up the spine, bypassing the left leg. On the next out-breath, alternate legs as you direct the breath to the left leg and into the floor. Now, engage only the left ankle, letting the engagement proceed up the leg and then the spine and—you guessed it—directing the next out-breath down the right leg. Continue this over and over, alternating legs.

As you continue this maneuver notice that a few different things are happening. First, as you direct your out-breath into one leg or the other, feel how the energy flowing into that leg shifts your body to the same side. Try your best not to influence how your body shifts; just let it happen on its own as it follows the breath. Notice how when the out-breath flows into one leg, it energizes that leg and that side becomes very stable, or grounded. When you start the progressive engagement from that foot and ankle up towards the hip, it accentuates that stability even more. Then notice how as you engage one leg, the other leg becomes lighter, and as you continue that engagement up through the spine, the opposite leg starts to elevate, along with the upper body.

Continue this side-to-side rhythm of BodyBreathing, allowing yourself to connect more deeply with these sensations. Feel grounding on one side and lightness on the other. Notice how the deeper you ground on one side, the lighter the other side feels as they are connected. On the next in-breath, as you start to engage your ankle, simultaneously push the same foot into the ground. Doing this will accentuate a lift of the opposite leg. This time, allow the lift to raise that foot off of the floor just a couple of inches, or (if that is uncomfortable for you) simply lift only the heel, keeping your toes on the ground for support. Do this very slowly at first and take time to let yourself experience the power of these shifting energy flows.

The next step (pun intended) is to allow your opposite foot to rise up as you engage and actively ground your leg on one side. This sequential engagement will in turn create more lightness and lift on the rising leg. As this happens, let the rising leg swing forward and take a very small step, a micro-step. As your leg swings forward and your foot lands on the floor, direct the next out-breath into that leg, allowing it to become the forward, grounded leg. This is the leg from which you will initiate the next in-breath. As you ground and engage this forward leg, the other leg will lighten and begin to rise. Accentuate this by raising your shoulders towards your ears as your back leg rises up and swings forward. When this leg lands, direct the out-breath into the new forward leg and integrate into the floor.

Is this starting to seem familiar? You are grounding yourself with each step and making yourself lighter with each breath. You are, as I like to say, levitating yourself across the room. Who else walks like this? Remember the toddler we discussed earlier? We are taking a lesson from our youth and returning to our roots. So, just as with Junior, this process requires a lot of your attention, and it will feel like you are learning how to walk all over again (which you are).

It is not unreasonable to spend 10 to 15 minutes a day on this practice alone. I have found this invaluable for my patients. It allows people to learn that they "can take it with them." What makes SitStandStroll so powerful is that it is portable. We are creating a background energy flow that will, in time, turn into our new HabitEnergy. This is how we are going to reclaim our youthful lightness. The more you do it, the easier it becomes.

Sit

Now that you have a sense of the Stand and Stroll elements of the practice, we will turn to the Sit pose. If you expect this to be the easy part, you may be surprised. To begin, sit in a firm chair. If you are sitting all the way back in your chair, leaning against the backrest, stop. This is not a healthy way to sit, and it is only beneficial to the physical therapist and orthopedic surgeon, as it will surely cause back problems in time that will send you to their offices. Instead, slide your body forward until you are sitting on the edge of your chair, far enough that you can freely rock your pelvis forward and plant your feet firmly on the floor. You may feel like you are going to fall off at first, but don't worry—you won't if you keep your feet firmly planted on the floor.

Determine if your body position is correct by placing your hand on the small of your back. Now rock your pelvis forward and back. When you rock back far enough you will feel these hard, spiny structures in the middle of your spine stick out. This means you are sitting back too far on your pelvis and that the curve in your spine is unhealthy. Next, rock your pelvis forward until those bony, spinous protrusions disappear. When that happens, you have tilted your pelvis far enough to create a healthy curve in your back. Now, simply lift your shoulders. Look down at your feet and check to see that your toes are pointed straight ahead.

With your feet firmly planted on the ground, let's BodyBreathe. Tighten the muscles in your ankles, then calves, and then around your thighs. Draw your belly button into your spine and squeeze the muscles around your lower, middle, and then upper back. Feel the in-breath as you fully engage your body from toe to head. Please be aware it is more difficult to appreciate the flow of your breath in the sitting position than it is in the standing position. Also note that if you are sitting too far back on your chair and your pelvic motion is restricted, it will be even more difficult. You may need to reposition yourself on your chair and start again. As we proceed with the out-breath, let the breath travel down your back, down your butt, then your thighs, calves, and through your feet into the floor. Start the in-breath all over again: ankles, calves, thighs, belly button, lower back, middle back, and upper back.

BodyBreathing in Sit feels very different than when we are standing because of the chair. The chair breaks the flow of energy, so in order to feel the breath clearly, our legs and lower back have to be very strong. I remember that when I started do this practice, I assumed because it was "chair yoga" it should be easier. Then came the realization that even sitting I needed to use my legs, and I was shocked at how weak mine were. So what did I do? I continued to reposition my body on my chair to get the required freedom and stability in my lower back and pelvis. I used the chair to my advantage. Instead of the chair making my posture weaker, I found a way to use the chair to make it stronger.

Let's try this: On your next in-breath, after exhaling completely, tighten your legs and, while you pull your belly button into your spine, curl your tailbone into the chair you are sitting on. This time, concentrate on keeping your legs engaged throughout both the in-breath and the out-breath. This will remain constant. As you exhale and the out-breath travels down the spine, notice how it instills strength into your spine and lower back. Holding on to the engagement of your legs, and now your lower back, at the end of the out-breath, actively push your pelvis into your seat, grounding your spine. Think of the chair as an extension of the floor. Notice how it creates a lift in your body, then squeeze the muscles around your lower, middle, and upper back (you should feel an in-breath as you do this). At the top of the in-breath, pause, and then start the out-breath and let it drain down your back into the chair as if it were the floor (remember, your legs are still engaged). Keeping your legs tight, once again by tightening the spinal muscles all the way up your back, feel the experience, and then guide the out-breath down your back into the chair.

Another variation: On the next out-breath, feel how integrated and aligned your body becomes. Keep that engagement, pause, and with your body engaged simply lift your chest and shoulders, noticing how the breath naturally fills your lungs. Exhale into the chair again and pause. Continue to repeat these actions and notice that you are working your body even while you are sitting in your chair. You are creating total engagement, using more and more of your body to breathe and align. Keep bringing your awareness to this process. Close your eyes and feel the breath as it flows up and down your spine. As you breathe in and out, let yourself feel whatever there is to feel in this moment. Imagine that this next breath you take will be the most important breath of your entire life, followed by the next breath, followed by the next....

Meditation

Meditation is an ancient practice for cultivating awareness. In every major religious or spiritual tradition, we find forms of meditation that vary in their approach but have a similar goal: to expand awareness and quiet the mind. These days, meditation is increasingly popular with people from all walks of life who have discovered its tremendous benefits for stress reduction, relaxation, and health. A 2007 study by the U.S. government found that nearly 9.4 percent of U.S. adults (more than 20 million people) had practiced meditation within the past 12 months. This simple form of meditation can assist you as you continue to cultivate your awareness of the energy flows we exploit in SitStandStroll. In order to guide the breath through the body in a new pattern, you need to be able to bring your awareness to this flow of energy. The daily practice of meditation, focused on the breath, can help to make this energy flow easily accessible on a daily basis.

Believe it or not, we have already begun the process of meditation: BodyBreathing. In fact, it is a moving meditation. Consider that anytime you pause to experience the breath, you are meditating, even if you are in motion. Meditation is simply focused awareness. Even as we move, we can be aware and meditative. Have you ever heard an athlete talk about when they are "in the zone"? This is a state where they can do no wrong. A batter can hit any pitch, and a pitcher can strike out any batter. Why is that? It is because they stop thinking in the usual sense and just are. No matter how fast the pitcher throws his fastball, a hitter "in the zone" will be able to see it clearly.

This is what SitStandStroll focuses on. What if we make everything we do, such as sitting, standing, or strolling, into a meditation? When our lives become meditative we live in the zone. This not only improves our health, but also adds a new dimension to our lives that can only be described by someone who meditates. I can tell you that any patient, family member, or friend who has taken my recommendation on meditation to heart and pursued the practice has always been overwhelmed with the benefits and in turn readily recommends it to all who will listen.

Getting Out of Our Own Way

The yoga teacher Sharon Gannon said, "You cannot do yoga. Yoga is your natural state. What you can do are yoga exercises, which may reveal to you where you are resisting your natural state." I think this is a very insightful comment, and one worth keeping in mind as you practice. When you discover areas of difficulty and resistance, it often feels as if you are trying to do something "unnatural." But this is only because it has become your habit to be out of alignment. Don't force your way through; relax, re-engage, and ground yourself, allowing the resistance to slowly release.

Yoga, as I have said, is often about getting out of your own way. By bringing awareness and engagement to our everyday movements, we are able to break the habit patterns that have formed in resistance to our natural state of health and wholeness. When we get out of our own way, we allow our bodies to heal themselves. This is why I often say that yoga is really not that mystical at all—it is common sense. When we stop making unhealthy choices and living toxic lifestyles, the natural healing energy that is present in our bodies can express itself.

Don't be hard on yourself if you don't always succeed in making healthy choices. A big part of yoga is recognizing when we make bad choices and bringing awareness to these moments so that we can become conscious of the alternative. The recognition is a victory in itself.

When we are in balance, a natural, healthy rhythm pulsates through our bodies and we feel good. The practice of yoga allows us to connect with that rhythm. When we are out of balance, our bodies, minds, and emotions are out of sync with nature, and we know there is something wrong. Through the lifestyle practices we learn in yoga, we are able to connect more profoundly to these deeper currents in our everyday lives so we can identify what it is that is bothering us. For many people, that kind of connection is only experienced in moments of heightened intensity. Perhaps you have felt it when engaging in some form of extreme sports, like downhill skiing, bungee-cord jumping, or waterskiing. At such times we feel more alive, more "in the flow" of the universe. Perhaps the birth of a child or falling in love has given you a taste of this deeper connection. Even tragic moments can have this effect because we are suddenly shocked into connecting more deeply with the preciousness of being alive. Whether it is a large-scale tragedy like September 11, 2001, or a personal loss, the experience is of waking up to a deeper and more meaningful relationship to life. When we practice yoga and create greater integration in our own being, we can cultivate that connection to our more subtle currents, not only during these peak experiences but during our everyday lives.

CHAPTER 9

Creating Healthy Eating Habits

"Let food be thy medicine, thy medicine shall be thy food."

—HIPPOCRATES

DIET IS PERHAPS the most contentious issue when it comes to our health. People do not want to give up their food despite the fact that it might be killing them. This is perhaps the best example of HabitEnergy I can think of. What is it about changing the way we eat that is so difficult? What is it about our food that leaves us so stuck in our ways that people are willing to die for it?

When Dr. Ornish conducted the Lifestyle Heart Trial, it was supposed to be about yoga. When the information went public, however, even though yoga was perhaps the biggest aspect of the program, it was rarely mentioned. All anyone talked about was the fact that it was vegan and low fat. This study officially launched our country into the low-fat craze in the early 1990s, which would not have been a bad thing if we had really followed the advice of Dr. Ornish. Instead we became experts at consuming low-fat junk food.

I remember watching Dr. Ornish debate Dr. Atkins, creator of the Atkins Diet, on television about the relative merits of the Atkins Diet versus a whole food, low fat, vegan diet. Diet is indeed an important aspect of our heart health, but it is not everything. In fact, in Dr.

Ornish's study, diet accounted for only 25 percent of the benefits, with the other 75 percent being equally divided between smoking cessation, exercise, and yoga, which included group support. But even though diet is not everything, it is an undeniably important step.

I think it is safe to say that the medical community will never agree on what is truly heart healthy because there are too many competing interests at stake, both economic and personal. Our diets are heavily influenced by our culture, family background, emotional states, psychological makeup, economic circumstances, and many, many other factors. These have created deeply ingrained HabitEnergies, making it difficult to make the necessary changes or even be able to see the wisdom of changing.

Remember, we are now working from an energy model. What we ultimately want to explore is the experience of nutrifying our bodies rather than just feeding it food. The experience of eating includes the decision process on what to eat, the actual preparation of the food, how we feel when we consume the food, and how to we feel after we eat, both physically and emotionally. As we work through the process, we discover that a good portion of what we eat is due to our emotions. Once we get past that hurdle we can navigate our options with greater ease.

The preparation and consumption of what we eat is more important than almost anything else that we do because it affects us on so many different levels. Yet, when it comes to food, we are probably less selective and less conscious about it than any other aspect of our lives. The most common complaints from my patients about dietary modification are that they do not have the time to prepare the food, it is hard to find recipes, it is too expensive, or their families won't support them. For most of us, every meal we consume is a toxic assault on our bodies. After we eat, our bodies have to mount an effort to protect our blood vessels and hearts from the poisons that we continuously consume. I often tell my patients that when we eat high fructose corn syrup, it is like rubbing sandpaper on the finish of your new car. It damages our bodies very slowly but surely.

The reality is that we are not even aware of what is happening and that things can be done differently. My intent is not to lay down the law about what you should and shouldn't eat; rather, it is to inform you of your options and the consequences of those options—both good and bad—so you can begin to make better choices in your everyday life. My hope is that when you are informed of the facts and make some changes, you will discover for yourself how delicious healthy food really is, how easy it is to prepare, and, above all, how good it makes you feel. You will begin to make better choices more and more frequently.

I know fully that there will be many who will disagree with my diet recommendations. What I ask is that you keep an open mind and see what works for you. I will show you how to take simple, manageable steps towards the ideal, slowly creating new and healthier eating habits. The good news is that every step you take will in and of itself bring enormous benefits in terms of your health and vitality.

The Ideal Diet

So what is the ideal diet? The ideal diet is a nondairy, whole-food, vegan diet such as Dr. Ornish recommended years ago. That means eliminating all animal products, including meat, eggs, and dairy products, such as milk, butter, cheese, and ice cream. This is not just my personal recommendation, or even just the opinion of holistic practitioners. One of the most respected diet studies ever conducted, the China-Oxford-Cornell Diet and Health Project, came to this same conclusion after studying the connection between diet, lifestyle factors, and disease mortality in 65 rural Chinese counties over a 25-year period. The study was described by the New York Times as the "most comprehensive large study ever undertaken of the relationship between diet and the risk of developing disease." In the bestselling The China Study, by T. Colin Campbell and Thomas M. Campbell II, the results confirmed that "People who ate the most animal-based foods got the most chronic disease.... People who ate the most plant-based foods were the healthiest and tended to avoid chronic disease." Citing more than 8,000 statistically significant cases, "These results could not be ignored."

If you really want to give your body the best chance at optimal health—and I know this is a tall order—it is my recommendation that you should give up meat and all animal products. In addition, I recommend eliminating all processed foods—the so-called "white foods," like white bread, pastas, white sugar, and so on—and replacing these with whole-grain alternatives. I also encourage eating plenty of vegetables and fruit as well as shifting to buying organic, locally-grown produce whenever possible. Also, do not consume genetically modified foods (GMOs) as they are not safe. I understand this may not seem realistic to many, but I am simply telling you what I have come to consider the ideal based on all the evidence available to me.

If these measures seem extreme to you, it is important to consider the alternatives. Would you really prefer to face open-heart surgery, or take more medications, than to simply change what you put on your dinner table? The hard truth is that most people and medical professionals seem only too happy to choose the former, as nonsensical as it seems. As Dr. Ornish writes, "I don't understand why asking people to eat a well-balanced vegetarian diet is considered drastic, while it is medically conservative to cut people open and put them on cholesterol lowering drugs for the rest of their lives."

There are a number of excellent heart healthy diet books on the market. My favorites are written by Dean Ornish, M.D., Joel Fuhrman, M.D., and Neal Barnard, M.D., because they are plant based and loaded with data that will help you understand why these recommendations have been made. There are other diets that will allow you to consume animal protein, including red meat, poultry, pork, seafood, and dairy. What is common to any meaningful diet is that processed foods be eliminated, especially high fructose corn syrup. I believe that it is our duty to boycott these products so that the producers stop making them as they are harming the public, especially our children. In addition, all artificial sweeteners should be eliminated as they also are harmful to our bodies. We should focus on whole foods that are locally grown without chemicals and avoid produce that is grown with pesticides or grown from genetically modified seeds. If you find it impossible to eliminate animal products, then l would limit them to less than 5 percent of your total food consumption.

Healthy Transitions

That being said, I know all too well that most people simply can't, or won't, do what I would recommend as an ideal. Besides our habits and preferences, many of us face financial limitations that dictate our food choices. Where we live and where we work also affect what is available to us. So the most important thing is to recognize where you are starting from and then begin to make transitions forward. Every positive change has an impact. If you decide to give up drinking sodas and start drinking water instead, that will have an impact on your weight and health. If you give up eating hot dogs and have a grilled chicken breast on a whole-grain bun instead, that will have an impact. It may not be ideal, but it is a genuine step in the right direction.

I don't believe in being overly rigid about diet. It is more important to keep the conversation going. After all, the goal is to live well, not just to survive. I had the opportunity to reflect on this recently when I invited two of my long-term patients who have been attending my reversal program to talk with me over dinner about the program and the impact it had had on their lives. While happy to talk about their experience, they refused my invitation to take them to dinner, insisting instead on taking me to one of their favorite Polish restaurants. When I looked at the menu, there was not really anything that would fit the requirements of the ideal diet I have just described. Since I follow that diet myself, I improvised and ordered a Greek salad without the cheese.

The evening was delightful, however, sharing both the culture and the zest for life that defined these two men. At one point, I tried a pierogi, which is a Polish potato dumpling—basically starch on starch. I joked to myself that it was restaurants like this that kept cardiologists like me in business. And yet the two men sitting at that table with me were doing well, having been my patients for 13 and 15 years, respectively. They had both made significant transitions that dramatically improved their health and had been practicing yoga with me every Monday for just as many years. Who am I to impose my beliefs on them? Their food choices were not necessarily what I would call ideal, but they were tempered by awareness and moderated in ways that before they met me would have been inconceivable. To their friends they were considered the "health nuts," doing yoga with their wacko heart doctor. The steps they each had taken were providing a strong foundation for further shifts to take place in the future.

Lightness of Being

One of the most important aspects of Healthful Evolutions is developing an awareness of yourself in a way you have never before experienced. This serves a vital role when it comes to dietary modification. An important part of changing your eating habits is becoming more aware of the effects of food on your body as well as your being. As you cultivate this newfound awareness and engagement, you will be able to discern the effects of your food choices on you. Rather than mindlessly consuming whatever is easiest and most comfortable, you may decide to change your eating habits, not just because you have been told it is good for you, but because it simply makes you feel better.

The digestive system, as we have discussed, has an energy flow of its own, and what we put into it affects the experience of that flow. The fact is that most of us in the West are used to overeating at breakfast, lunch, dinner, and often in between. Have you ever noticed that when you overeat, you feel bloated and heavy? Do you notice that you eat just because the food is there and you "want to finish your plate"?

It feels good momentarily, but soon all that is left is an unpleasant sense of heaviness and lethargy. Experiment with eating less and replacing the heavy, greasy foods on your plate with fresh vegetables or salad. You will notice that you start to experience a lightness of being and discover an unexpected wellspring of energy that had previously been dampened down by overeating.

This is where the HabitEnergy comes in. Just because you don't feel full doesn't mean you haven't eaten enough. For an experiment, the first time you want to attempt a conscious change, eat 50 percent of what you usually eat and then stop. Walk away from the table and observe. Notice the feeling that tells you that you have not eaten enough is just another example of a HabitEnergy you have cultivated over the years.

This is a particularly common sensation if you are a meat eater, especially if you are a red-meat eater. I remember as a child when my mother, in an attempt to bring diversity to the dinner table, would serve fish. After dinner, it seemed as if we had not had eaten yet. It wasn't until some meat or poultry was consumed that I was satisfied. So I am under no illusions about what you are going through. The yoga, if you will, is to observe ourselves as we experience the uneasiness that is brought about by this HabitEnergy and what we do to deal with it. They say it takes about 40 days for a "new" habit to replace an old habit. This is when our BodyBreathing comes into play. My advice, in such challenging moments, is to BodyBreathe.

Not in an urgent or panicked way—just a very calm slow in-breath, followed by a long, slow, deliberate out-breath. As you focus on the breathing you "see" the sensations in your body as they are happening to you. At this point, watch yourself deal with this difficult issue. Instead of it being you with the "problem," imagine it is someone else you know and love deeply, like a child, grandchild, spouse, or parent. What would you say to them? Would you tell them they are no good and can't do anything with their lives, or would you offer them encouragement, love, and compassion, cheering them on in their efforts? This can offer great insight into how our own internal dialogue influences our outcomes.

As you continue to bring awareness to your eating habits, you will begin to notice how much you think about food. I remember when I fasted for the first time. For four days I consumed nothing but water and some supplements. I was amazed at how much I thought about food. It made me realize how much food dominates our lives.

In time, and with continued practice, food will not dominate your life as much. Realize that when you are not thinking about food you can be thinking about something else. As you do, you will create space in your consciousness for many other things, which will allow you to connect more deeply with the energy of the life-force within yourself that will free you of this HabitEnergy.

Awareness increases your freedom of choice, releasing you from the relentless momentum of old, unhealthy HabitEnergies and enabling you to decide to go in a different direction. As you begin to make healthier choices and observe the results, you will find your preferences begin to change. Foods you once loved and thought you could never give up will start to be distasteful to you as you learn to associate them not only with the short-term pleasure of eating them, but with the heaviness, lethargy, and ill health that they lead to in the long term. Foods that you might have been indifferent to in the past will become more attractive as you recognize and appreciate the vitality and lightness in your being you feel after eating them. Allow space for your tastes to change. After all, if your favorite foods are killing you, something is not right. It is time for some new favorites.

People tend to think of diets as being about self-deprivation and willpower, but they are actually much more about education and awareness. Most of us simply don't know how to make better food choices, or how to prepare healthy foods in ways that are tasty as well as nutritious. For the past couple of years, I have been getting together with my good friend, vegetarian chef George Vutetakis, to run a series of workshops called "Food is Medicine." We teach people about a plant-based diet and show them how to prepare meals for themselves. It is always such a joy to see the surprise and delight on the faces of the participants when they discover how good the food can taste! If you check out his website, you will be amazed at the number of extremely delicious, healthy options that exist: www. thevegetarianguy.com.

So try making your first transition today. It doesn't matter if it's a small one, so long as it's a step in the right direction. Pay attention to how it makes you feel. Changing your diet doesn't have to be all about giving up what you want. It can be about learning to want things you never would have imagined you would be attracted to. Take the first step now and you may surprise yourself with where you end up.

EPILOGUE

A Life of Gratitude

WE STARTED OUT talking about heart disease, and we ended up with a new way to stand, breathe, and, most importantly, a new way to look at the world. Change is difficult, but only if we think that we are depriving ourselves. I don't know why it is so easy for some people to quit smoking on the day of their heart attack while the week before it would have been impossible to consider. Changing our outlook is perhaps the most important change we can make. By engaging in a building process rather than an exercise in deprivation, lifestyle modification is not a punishment; it becomes your passion. This is the ultimate Healthful Evolution.

My promise to you is that all of this will help you reverse and prevent your heart disease. If you commit 25 percent, you will get a 25 percent benefit, and if you commit 75 percent—you get the idea. What we are doing is changing the way our bodies react to life. When we behave one way, one set of chemicals is released into our bloodstreams, and when we behave another way, another set is released. We actually have more control over this than we know. Healthful Evolutions is dedicated to helping you take those very first steps so that you can experience these changes for yourself. Most importantly, what I want for you is to live a better life.

As we grow older, we may feel we have been cursed by challenges like heart disease and other illnesses. It is all too easy to feel as if life is against us, our days are numbered, and things are only going to get worse from here on out. This attitude, however, while understandable, is not going to do us any good. In fact, it causes our bodies to flood our bloodstream with unhealthy chemicals that actually accelerate the disease process.

Believe it or not, this attitude was learned and cultivated that same way we learned to stand and breathe in a dysfunctional way. These ideas are part of what I believe is the most overlooked energy flow, our thoughts. And in the same way that we are able to change the energy flow in our bodies and blood vessels, we can also change the energy flow of our thoughts. To use a common cliché, we need to assume that our cup is half full, not half empty. This attitude is something best practiced on a daily basis.

I often find it challenging to embrace a positive attitude, so I have adopted the simple exercise of listing all the things I am grateful for. Gratitude is a powerful and healing energy that banishes negativity in a miraculous way. I recently read a book by a man who wrote a "thank you" note every day for a year. I was blown away by the idea. What a powerful practice!

It makes perfect sense. When we start to put our attention on the things we have to feel grateful for instead of the things we feel bad about, we change the energy flow in our lives, our minds, and our beings. Spiritual teachers tell us, "Where attention goes, energy flows." Our reality focuses on the things we spend the most time on. If every day we focused on what is wrong, then that is where we are going to spend all of our time. If we focus on ten things we are grateful for, however, our energy will shift, and we will begin to lead significantly happier and healthier lives.

I am not saying that you should deny the difficulties and problems in life, and it is perfectly understandable that none of us wants to suffer, get sick, or grow old. But in each and every one of these challenges we can find reasons for gratitude. We can be grateful for the opportunities they present for us to grow, to transform, to become more conscious, and even to change our unhealthy lifestyles to healthy lifestyles. Out of adversity comes greatness! We can be grateful that we have woken up from our unconsciousness and are now changing our HabitEnergies before it is too late.

I like to take the view that we are living in abundant times. In spite of the harsh economic conditions that prevail during the writing of this book, I believe that there are many valuable lessons to be learned. If we continue to look for the good in things, that is what we are going to find. I suggest that you consider making a practice of looking for the positive in everything you do in the same spirit of writing a thank-you note every day. In time, that is how your brain will naturally operate, as it will have created a new HabitEnergy.

Examine your thoughts. Note when you are able to be kind to yourself with an uplifting internal conversation. Also note when your thoughts want to punish you, when they are critical and demeaning. First and foremost, realize they are just thoughts, they are not you, and thoughts can be changed (they are, after all, HabitEnergy). As you do that, notice how you feel inside. Sound familiar? It is the same as when we want to eat mindlessly. So simply pause, recognize it, and do your BodyBreathing, no matter where you are or what you are doing. Rather than getting down on yourself for having a negative thought, celebrate the fact that you noticed! Then replace the negative thought with a positive thought. At first it will feel awkward, but it will quickly become much easier, and you will slowly but surely form a new healthy HabitEnergy.

This is another way of living and a very powerful yoga practice. When we consider how much of the conversation in our heads has been devoted to failure, it is amazing that we have made it this far. Imagine the possibilities if we cheered for ourselves with the same love and compassion that we seem to save for our special loved ones.

Don't we deserve the same level of joy and happiness that we desire for them?

The reality is that it is all there for us. Eckhart Tolle tells a story in The Power of Now about a beggar who sits on a box for thirty years without knowing it has been filled with gold all along. That is our own condition. Our bodies want to heal themselves, and all we have to do is respect and align with the universal laws of nature to reap the rewards. Surrender yourself to the endless possibilities that are yet to be. No one really knows what is in their future, no matter how much they plan for it, and you are no exception. Perhaps your life is actually perfect and everything that has happened up to now was meant to bring you to this exact moment. And perhaps this is a perfect moment that is to be followed by another perfect moment, and another, and another. And yes, it is time to breathe.

ENDNOTES

i   Dean Ornish, *Dr. Dean Ornish's Program for Reversing Heart Disease* (New York: Random House, 1995) p. xix

ii   Tom Rath, Jim Harter, James K. Harter, *Well Being* (Washington, DC: Gallup Press, 2010) p. 87

iii   Larry Dossey, *The Extraordinary Healing Power of Ordinary Things* (New York: Random House, 2007) p. 17

iv   Larry Dossey, *The Extraordinary Healing Power of Ordinary Things* (New York: Random House, 2007) p. 17

v   See the WHO website: http://www.who.int/suggestions/faq/en/index.html

vi   Henry Miller, *A Devil In Paradise* (New York: New American Library, 1961)

vii   *Astadala Yogamala, The Collected Works of BKS Iyengar* (New Delhi: Allied Publishers Limited)

viii   Jane E. Brody, "Huge Study Of Diet Indicts Fat And Meat," *New York Times* May 8, 1990

ix   T. Colin Campbell and Thomas M. Campbell, *The China Study* (Dallas, TX: BenBella Books, 2006) p. 7

x   John Robbins, *Healthy Heart, Healthy Life* (Newburyport, MA: Conari Press, 2010) p. 25

ABOUT THE AUTHOR

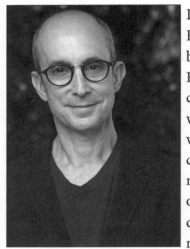 DR. MICHAEL DANGOVIAN, DO, FACC, is an integrative, yoga-based, board certified cardiovascular specialist. His evidence based, clinical practice combines the best of the traditional western medical model with ancient wisdom of the East, forming what is currently referred to as integrative medicine. His unique approach focuses on treating the cause of the many chronic diseases that plague our society today, most notably heart disease, rather than simply treating the symptoms of chronic disease with medications. Dr. Dangovian is the owner of Healthy Heart & Vascular, PLLC and is the founder and medical director of the Wellness Training Institute.

For more information visit
http://www.healthyheartandvascular.com *and*
http://www.wellnesstraininginstitute.com

INDEX